A User's Guide To Chinese Medicine

NEIL KINGHAM

Copyright © 2013 by Neil Kingham

All rights reserved. This book or any portion thereof may not be reproduced or used in any manner whatsoever without the express written permission of the author except for the use of brief quotations in a book review.

First Printing, 2013
ISBN 978-1493720439

www.neilkingham.com

Information in this book is not meant as a substitute for the advice of your own physician or other medical professional. This information should not be used to diagnose, treat or attempt to prevent any disease. If you are suffering from any ailment that may require medical attention, seek advice from a qualified professional. If you are currently taking medication or under medical care for any illness or ailment, do not begin to consume herbs or supplements without informing your doctor.

To Molly

Contents

Authors Introduction 8

Section 1 - Introducing Chinese Medicine

1. What Is Chinese Medicine? *13*
   Different Paradigms *14*
   The Westernisation Of Chinese Medicine *16*

2. The 5 Branches Of Chinese Medicine *21*

3. Holistic Medicine And the Causes Of Disease *25*
   Human Qi And The Organ Correspondences *26*
   The Causes Of Disease *28*

4. Using Chinese Medicine - 3 Steps To Radiant Health *35*

Section 2 - Diagnosis

5. Step 1 Of 3 - Diagnose Energetic Imbalance *41*
   Diagnostic Theories *43*
   Diagnostic Techniques *44*

6. The Main Disharmonies *49*
   Qi Deficiency *51*
   Yang Deficiency *52*
   Blood Deficiency *54*
   Yin Deficiency *56*
   Jing Deficiency *58*
   Full Cold *60*
   Full Heat *61*

Qi Stagnation *62*
Blood Stagnation *64*
Dampness *65*
Phlegm *67*
Wind (External Invasions) *68*
Internal Wind *69*
Patterns Case Study - Janet *70*

7. The Organs *72*
Organ Imbalances *74*
Lungs *76*
Spleen *79*
Heart *82*
Kidneys *85*
Pericardium And San Jiao *88*
Liver *91*
Organs Case Study - Janet Revisited *94*
Mixed Patterns *95*

Section 3 - Treatment

8. **Step 2 Of 3 - Treat Current Conditions** *101*
The 5 Branches Of Chinese medicine *101*
Choosing A Practitioner *102*

9. **Acupuncture And Tui Na - The Channels And Acupoints** *105*
The Energetic Body *105*
Acupuncture *109*
Tui Na *114*

10. **Nutrition And Herbalism - The Energetic properties Of Plants** *119*
Energetics vs Chemical Constituents *119*
Dietary Therapy / Nutrition *121*

Herbalism *125*

11. T'ai Chi and Chi Kung *129*
Exercising The Qi *129*

12. Supplementary Treatments *134*
Moxa *134*
Cupping *137*
Gua Sha *138*
Other Supplementary Treatments *139*

13. After Your Treatment *140*

Section 4 - Maintenance, Prevention And 'Nourishing Life'

14. Step 3 Of 3 - Cultivate Radiant Health *145*

15. Yang Sheng - Nourishing Life *148*

Section 5 - Final Thoughts And Resources

16. Putting It All Together *157*
Case Study - Simon *158*

Glossary *161*
Resources *167*

Authors Introduction

The various therapies and treatments that make up 'Chinese Medicine' have become very popular in the UK and elsewhere in the Western world, but they are often misunderstood, and can seem arcane, mystical and baffling.

While there are quite a few books that serve as 'beginners guides' to Chinese Medicine, they are often very heavy on theory, and not aimed at someone actually receiving Chinese medicine treatment.

In my clinics, when I have been talking to patients and clients about their treatments, explaining how they worked, and why I was doing certain things and not others, I have often been asked if I could recommend a book along similar lines. As I didn't know of one, I couldn't. So now, after quite a few years, and some 'gentle persuasion' from some of those same clients and patients, here is that book.

This is a guide to the varied methods and techniques that can make up Chinese Medicine. It is for those who are currently having, or are considering having, some kind of treatment themselves. It will explain the process from beginning to end, from diagnosis, through to treatment and then to maintenance and improved well-being, a process which I call 'The 3 Steps To Radiant Health.'

This is also a book for t'ai chi or chi kung students, complementary or mainstream health practitioners, or other interested parties who would like to understand more about the practice of Chinese Medicine.

The theory of Chinese Medicine takes many years to learn, and uses a number of terms and concepts that will be unfamiliar to the average Western reader. Rather than go into these in massive detail, I have chosen to abbreviate and simplify where possible, focusing on what you need to know to understand what a treatment entails.

For instance, in the first main section of this book, about diagnosis, I have not spent long describing the nature and functions of the substances and energies such as Qi, Blood, Yin and Yang – whole books could be (and have been) written about the nature of Qi alone – instead I have talked in terms of disharmonies, such as 'Qi deficiency' or 'Damp-Heat' which are the diagnostic terms that are used in clinical practice. These are the kinds of terms your practitioner will use when speaking to you.

I have limited the use of Chinese words where possible. There are 2 systems for 'romanising' Chinese words (i.e. writing them using our Roman alphabet), and I have not stuck to one or the other, but used whichever is in more common usage – for instance a few paragraphs above using 't'ai chi' instead of 'taiji' and 'chi kung' instead of 'qi gong' but 'qi' instead of 'chi' – You can use the glossary in the back of the book to help you to decipher different spellings or other Chinese terms, if you encounter them elsewhere.

I hope that you enjoy this book and find it useful, and that it gives you an insight into the world of Chinese medicine, and some ideas about how you can most effectively use this ancient healing system in your own life. I welcome your feedback and questions – you can contact me via my website at www.neilkingham.com

Neil Kingham, Sept 2013
South Wales

SECTION 1

Introducing Chinese Medicine

CHAPTER ONE

What Is Chinese Medicine?

The practice of Chinese medicine pre-dates written records, and nobody knows exactly when or how it started. Hieroglyphs dating from approximately 1000 BC, during the Chinese Shang Dynasty, showed evidence of acupuncture, and bronze needles have been excavated from ruins dating from this era but in fact it is likely that Chinese medicine was being practised some time before that.

What we do know is that over at least 3000 years, the Chinese have developed an understanding of humankind, and the functions and dysfunctions of the body, mind and spirit that lead to the development of a system of medicine that has served billions.

In modern times Chinese medicine has spread around the globe, and becomes more and more popular in the West as people look for more holistic and natural methods of health care and treatment.

The most important thing to understand about Chinese medicine is that it is based on a fundamentally different way of looking at health and illness than Scientific Western medicine. In the most basic terms, Chinese medicine is a medicine of energetics. That is, it is concerned with our energetic body, our Qi. As you will see, this makes the practice of Chinese medicine an entirely different undertaking to that of Western medicine.

Different Paradigms

Chinese medicine is holistic, while modern Western medicine is reductionist – Where Western medicine continually drills down into more specific and smaller areas, Chinese medicine builds up an overall picture of the whole person. Western medicine looks at systems, organs and diseases in isolation, and Chinese medicine looks at the inter-relations between all aspects of the person and environment. Western medicine tries to treat the symptoms of disease, while Chinese medicine always seeks to understand and treat the root cause of a condition.

The important thing to remember is that modern Western medicine and traditional Chinese medicine are worlds apart. They have incompatible ways of looking at health, illness, and indeed the whole of existence. This doesn't mean that one is wrong, or one is better than the other. However, what it does mean is that you can't mix the two.

In the Western paradigm, the experience of the patient is not given much importance. Only measurable, observable phenomena are given any weight, for instance lab tests, x-rays and MRI scans. Because they are objective, they are seen to reveal the 'truth' behind the condition. This approach automatically takes the person out of the picture, not only disregarding what could be important diagnostic information, but also downgrading and de-personalising the provision of healthcare. What 'you' think or feel, or your own ideas about your condition, become irrelevant.

You become a machine with a malfunctioning part, and the doctor becomes the technician whose job it is to fix the machine. This is achieved by finding the one specific cause of the problem, and fixing it. These doctor-technicians have knowledge that is deep, but narrow - they are very highly trained but only in a very specific area. This can be useful on the occasions when a condition or illness falls very definitely in only that one specific area, but given the complex nature of the interrelationships between different systems and conditions, this is a rare occurrence.

In this approach, the doctor has all the knowledge and power, and you have none. The body's self-healing power is almost completely disregarded, and it is the doctor who applies a healing intervention (such as drugs or surgery) from the outside.

In contrast, Chinese medicine takes a broad view, in which the personal experience of life and health is vital, and objective and subjective measures are combined to create a wide-ranging understanding of a person's current state of being. These subjective feelings, instincts and observations make up an important part of the overall pattern that describes exactly what kinds of imbalances might be present.

No one specific cause is sought, as complex and dynamic systems like a human being do not follow a simple linear route of one cause leading to one effect. Instead there is a complex 'web' of influences, signs and symptoms which must be considered as a whole. This complex system is always in motion, always changing, and yet always maintaining balance and equilibrium. It's when balance and equilibrium fail, that disease and illness occur.

Chinese medicine trusts the wisdom of the individual, and the doctor or practitioner will work with you as an equal – you share the knowledge and the power. The healing power of the body is respected and encouraged, and the healing comes not from without, but from within.

The Western approach to health separates out all the different processes that makes us who we are, and does not acknowledge the inter-relations between different parts of the body, mind and spirit in the same way that Chinese medicine does. Only in Western medicine could it make sense to have doctors of the body and separate doctors of the mind! In Chinese medicine, the mind and body are inseparable. Your thoughts, feelings and emotions are a part of you just as much as your body is, and play just as important a role in your health and quality of life. Changes to the body effect mind and emotions, and changes in emotions and thought effect the body. There is no way to separate these different facets of life.

The Westernisation of Chinese Medicine

The standard model of Chinese medicine taught and practised both in China and in the West is called 'Traditional Chinese Medicine' or 'TCM'. Ironically, given its name, this style of practice was formulated as recently as the 1960s by Chairman Mao's Communist Party. It was created by a process of standardisation, which drew together the many and varied roots, styles and approaches within Chinese medicine across the country, and formed for the first time a single syllabus that could be taught and practised across China.

As with any kind of standardisation process, some things were gained in this process, and some were lost. The motivations behind the creation of TCM were largely political, and much of what was lost was the spiritual side of the medicine. The mental and emotional aspects were also down-played, and the focus was put on physical conditions and treatments.

This began a gradual process of 'Westernisation' of Chinese medicine in China. The Chinese were keen to be (and be seen to be) 'modern', and embraced Western medicine, to the extent that reductionist principles began to replace traditional holistic ideas.

I'm not one of those practitioners who knocks Western medicine – it is a wonderfully advanced body of knowledge and expertise which has saved and continues to save many lives. As I often say, if I get run over by a bus, please take me to A&E, not to my acupuncturist!

But in modern China, while there are still some very traditional, holistic practitioners, many Chinese doctors are essentially practising Chinese medicine within a Western framework. I even know of so called 'traditional' Chinese doctors who are practising acupuncture, who say that they don't believe in Qi!

Chinese hospitals will normally have both Western and Traditional departments, and will often incorporate acupuncture, tui na, herbs and other traditional methods alongside modern Western treatments. However, there are political, financial and societal pressures to favour Western treatments. I have spent time in Chinese hospitals, and many traditional doctors that I have spoken to predict that traditional treatments will not last much longer in hospital settings, because of the financial incentives that the hospitals received for prescribing Western medication.

An example of the Westernisation process is the increasingly popular method of analysing Chinese herbs using Western techniques, i.e. to look at the chemical constituents of a herb. However, the knowledge gained from this analysis is only useful in a Western framework, and cannot really be incorporated into the traditional understanding of the herb.

For instance, if you have your 'Chinese' hat on, a patient may have a diagnosis of Heat in the Heart. The treatment in this case is to clear heat from the Heart. There are specific herbs, as well as acupuncture points, that will do this for you. (More on these kinds of Chinese diagnoses later)

So knowing that a herb has the effect of clearing heat from the Heart is important, but knowing that the same herb contains certain levels of iron, fibre and vitamins, and specific phyto-nutrients and other chemicals is irrelevant. This is mixing up 2 different paradigms, in a way that benefits neither.

And on the other end of things – from the patient's point of view – it's a similar story. One of my most enduring memories from my travels in China is from about 10 years ago, when I was chatting to a young Chinese man, in his late teens or early twenties, over dinner. He was very interested that me and my friend, two Westerners, were in China to study acupuncture, and wondered about our motivations.

Once we had chatted for a while he asked me "so, what is it that acupuncture does?" Slightly confused, I asked him to restate the question. To my amazement, he didn't have a clue about what acupuncture was used for, and had never had it himself. Once we started discussing it, he told me that he thought that probably very few people his age had ever had acupuncture either.

When I asked him why, his answer was very revealing – he said that the younger generations were quite aware that Western medication had side effects, but they would rather go ahead and risk the side-effects because they were all busy and didn't have time to go for regular acupuncture appointments!

So with doctors less likely to recommend traditional treatments, and patients less likely to ask, the situation in China is that traditional medicine is dropping out of the mainstream. In a perfect balance of Yin and Yang, as it becomes less popular in its homeland, it becomes ever more popular in the West, with the ironic situation that many Western practitioners are more 'traditional' than their Chinese counterparts!

However, Western practitioners of Chinese medicine can fall into the trap of ' Westernisation' of Chinese medicine particularly easily, and many acupuncturists, herbalists and others pay lip service to holistic principles, but fail to grasp the 'big picture' of Chinese medicine as it has traditionally been practised. And missing this 'big picture', in my view, is missing the whole essence and power of this wonderful system.

And I'm not alone. More recently a new term, 'Classical Chinese Medicine' has been adopted. This is an approach to Chinese medicine which is rooted in the classic texts, that seeks to retain the holistic nature of the discipline, and does not deny the role of mental, emotional and spiritual sides of ourselves. It puts back into TCM what was removed by Mao's party, goes back to the roots of the medicine, and resists its 'Westernisation'.

There are advocates of this Classical Chinese Medicine approach in China, and also in the world at large, and I believe that it is these people that will be responsible for keeping the true nature of this medicine alive.

CHAPTER 2

The 5 Branches Of Chinese Medicine

Under the umbrella of 'Chinese medicine' are five main therapies, which are acupuncture, herbalism, tui na massage, t'ai chi / chi kung and dietary therapy / nutrition. Together, they form a complete system for health care, treatment of disease and personal cultivation and development.

These 5 Branches are united by a shared understanding of human health and illness based on the interplay between the different systems and energies that make up a human being. Although each branch uses a different method for treatment, the diagnostic process and the language and theories used to describe the current state of health or illness are the same for all five.

Although you may think of Chinese medicine as a treatment for illness, these arts are also very powerful tools for maintaining health and well-being, and preventing disease and illness. Indeed, they have always been used for this purpose, and to help to bring us into the highest possible state of physical, mental, emotional and spiritual well-being, which is sometimes called 'radiant health'. Using the 5 branches of Chinese medicine for self cultivation in this way is part of what is know as 'yang sheng' or 'nourishing life' – I explore this idea in more detail in Section 4.

These 5 Branches were always meant to work together, and the ancient Chinese doctors were masters of all five arts. This made them supremely flexible, and gave them the ability to tailor treatment precisely to each individual. In the UK, and most Western countries, there are many acupuncturists, Chinese herbalists and t'ai chi teachers, some tui na practitioners, and a few people working with Chinese nutritional therapy, but often these disciplines are practised in isolation.

As I have described, modern Western medicine likes to look for a singular cause of an illness, like a mechanic looking for the broken part of a machine. Once the broken part is found, it can be fixed or replaced. Chinese medicine, in contrast, takes a systems approach, and looks for overall imbalances. There is rarely a single cause, but rather a number of contributing factors, and these all need to be considered and addressed in the treatment plan. The complex nature of many modern illnesses and conditions, particularly chronic and degenerative conditions, makes this all the more important. This is where a flexible approach to treatment that does not rely on just one or two therapies is so useful.

The 'Life Stresses Pressure Gauge'

To illustrate this concept, imagine that you have a simple dial gauge that measures all the stresses and difficulties you have in your life. A needle on the gauge moves up and down as these pressures and difficulties come and go. A red line marked on the gauge shows the point where the pressure is too much, and illness begins.

At any given time there will be a number of things going on in your life that are contributing to the overall 'pressure', but for the sake of argument, lets imagine that there are three main pressures – work stress, poor diet and difficulty sleeping. These have built up to the point where the pressure gauge is very high, and has gone past the red line. You feel highly stressed, and are getting a lot of headaches, and your doctor tells you your blood pressure is up.

The Western options for treating your high blood pressure and headaches would probably be pain-killers and blood pressure tablets. These may or may not take the symptoms away, they certainly would not deal with any of the underlying problems. The Chinese approach would be to look at the whole person, and identify any imbalances or areas of difficulty, and treat the whole system. In this case, for instance, acupuncture or tui na could help to bring down stress levels and improve sleep – thus helping to get at the root of the problem.

But we could do more. Even with acupuncture and tui na the work stress is still there, and the diet is still bad. These are important contributing factors (and two thirds of the 'pressure' shown by the Life Stresses Pressure Gauge.) So a more integrated approach would include learning some stress-reduction and relaxation techniques to do at home to help you sleep, and maybe an 'emergency' de-stressing technique for use at times of particularly high stress.

Alongside the acupuncture or tui na treatment, this would effectively help you to cope with your work stresses, and help you sleep. Some advice about alterations to your diet will help to bring down the last third of the pressure gauge, moving the needle well down below the red line, and restoring health and well-being.

This also illustrates the problem with only sticking to one kind of treatment or therapy. Let's say you'd realised that your diet wasn't great, and you had gone to see a nutritional therapist for advice. With the correct guidance you could turn your diet around, and start to eat really well. This would certainly leave you feeling a lot better in many ways. However, it only deals with one of the three 'life pressures' – it does little or nothing to address your work stresses or sleeping problems. The trap here is to get fixated on diet. If improving your diet made you feel better, improving it more must make you feel even better, right?

Not necessarily. Once you've made the big change from not eating well to eating well, then any further improvements in diet will really be fine-tuning, and any improvements in health and well-being will only be incremental. If the pressure gauge is still above the red line, you need to address the two other big 'pressure' factors in your life. In this example, getting caught up in constantly fine-tuning your diet will not bring you the health goals that you're looking for.

This is an over-simplified example, but I hope it gives you an idea of a much more holistic and integrated approach to treatment that uses more than one branch of treatment, more in keeping with Classical Chinese values. For me, this is the strength and the heart of Chinese medicine.

CHAPTER 3

Holistic Medicine, And The Causes Of Disease

According to traditional Chinese thought, everything is composed of and exists because of Qi (sometimes spelled 'chi', and pronounced 'chee') In its widest sense, Qi accounts for all life, all inanimate objects, and all of the relationships within and between everything in the universe. By understanding the forms and actions of Qi we can understand ourselves, and the world around us.

Because Qi is everywhere, and everything is composed of Qi, a human being is not seen as a distinct unit separate from its surroundings. We are constantly taking in Qi, and giving it out. We interact with our environments and the other people around us on both gross and subtle levels all the time. Put simply, we are connected to everything, and everything is connected to us.

With this basic idea in mind, it can be seen that Chinese medicine must be holistic - the opposite approach to conventional Western medicine which is reductionist. Western medicine focuses in tightly on a specific organ, structure, or system, trying to get at the one individual thing that is causing the problem. Chinese medicine, in contrast, takes a wider view – It goes bigger and wider, taking in not only the specifics of the current problem but also many other aspects of the persons health and overall well-being.

Because everything is connected, nothing can be understood about a person without also understanding all the relevant influences and connections, which means understanding the internal and external environment in which the problem presents itself.

Human Qi, and the Organ Correspondences

Although the Qi of every person is a part of the Qi of the universe, in order to come to sensible and workable conclusions about an illness or disease, it is the Qi of the individual which the practitioner of Chinese Medicine is most concerned with. The 'external' Qi from the environment is also important as part of the overall picture, in as much as it effects and influences the personal Qi.

We divide the Qi of a human being into many types, depending on its role and functions. For instance, we talk of the Qi of the organs (Lung Qi, Bladder Qi, Heart Qi etc.) and we also talk of types of Qi with specific functions – for instance the Wei Qi protects the body from outside influences, and can be related to the concept of the immune system. The way the different types of Qi in the body influence and effect each other is very important to understanding health and illness.

At the level of the organs, we can say that organ Qi is a way of describing the function of the organs. So problems breathing, with wheezing and coughing may be described as a weakness or disharmony of Lung Qi.

In addition, the Qi of the organs corresponds to different colours, flavours, emotions, sounds, seasons, and many other things. These correspondences describe patterns in the functioning of Qi, and the connections between different aspects of our lives.

For instance, The emotion associated with the Lungs is grief or sadness, so a person with weak Lung Qi may be particularly prone to feeling sad. The Lung Qi may also be injured after a period of grief, for instance a bereavement, leading to respiratory problems. The season associated with the Lungs is Autumn, which means that conditions of the Lung Qi often appear at this time of year.

These might seem like arbitrary connections, but I have found them clinically useful and accurate on very many occasions. They are a tool that helps us to see the connection between the physical, mental, emotional and spiritual aspects of our lives, which can otherwise sometimes seem to be quite separate from each other.

The Causes Of Disease

With the inter-connectedness of different aspects of Qi, and the holistic nature of this medicine in mind, disease can be seen as a disruption to the system caused by some factor or factors which have broken the harmonious network of interactions and introduced imbalance.

These imbalancing factors are the causes of disease and illness and they are broadly broken down into three kinds - External, Internal and Miscellaneous.

External Causes

The External causes of disease account for influences on our health that arise from the environment. They are also called 'climatic factors' or 'external evils', and they are:

- Heat
- Wind
- Dampness
- Dryness
- Cold
- Summer Heat

Heat is stimulating and makes the Qi move fast and recklessly. If you have pathogenic Heat you feel hot, may have red skin, and can be irritable or angry.

Pathogenic Wind is unpredictable, and causes movements such as shaking or tremors, especially in the extremities, just as wind in the environment is also unpredictable, and makes things move and shake.

If you have Dampness you may feel that a heavy fog has settled inside you, weighing you down. Dampness slows down and stagnates the Qi, leading to lethargy, and there may be sticky secretions such as catarrh.

Dryness is pretty self-explanatory, and leads to dry skin or mouth, dry cough and dry stools.

The symptoms of Cold are also quite obvious - Cold causes a feeling of coldness, and a desire for heat, and can cause constricting pain.

Finally Summer Heat is a traditional term, said to occur only in the Summer, and can occur after prolonged exposure to the hot sun. Signs include a sudden high fever, sweating, red skin and thirst.

Internal Causes

The Internal causes of disease reflect the role of the emotions on health. Because emotions can be hard to categorise, and because different emotions are closely related, there have been a number of attempts over the years to label the different emotions, leading to the most common currently used list of the '7 Emotions':

- Joy
- Anger
- Pensiveness
- Sorrow
- Fear
- Fright
- Grief

The changing flow of emotions is a natural part of human

life, and it is certainly not the *experience* of emotions that causes illness. However, when emotions become disrupted or irregular, when their expression is prevented, or when any one emotion becomes excessive or deficient, then this can easily cause illness.

This is one of the important traditional causes of disease that has been given a reduced level of importance in modern TCM. Although the theory remains part of modern teaching, it is not seen to have as much clinical relevance as it once did.

However, in modern times the role of the emotions in overall health is actually of great significance. With advances in hygiene, improved nutrition and living conditions, we are less prone to serious contagious diseases and the influence of the elements, and more and more of our health problems come instead from emotional pressures, which we label with the broad term 'stress'.

This common-place 'stress' effects all of us in the modern world, and has been shown to have a wide range of debilitating effects on health and human functioning. I don't believe it's an exaggeration to say that stress is the main health problem facing us in the 'developed' world today.

This brings the Internal Causes of disease to the fore once again, and makes working in the realm of the emotions an important part of a Chinese Medicine practitioner's role.

Miscellaneous Causes

These are the causes which are 'neither internal nor external', and they include a wide range of different kinds of disease-causing influences and lifestyle factors.

When it comes to aspects of lifestyle that are contributing to poor health, there are two approaches to treatment - Using therapies to reduce the impact of the lifestyle factor, where changing lifestyle is not possible or desirable, and lifestyle coaching and guidance, to work together to uncover and understand the impact of lifestyle choice on health, and make changes where possible.

The miscellaneous causes of disease are:

- Constitution
- Nutrition
- Occupation
- Overwork
- Sex and Relationships
- Trauma
- Parasites and Poisons
- Iatrogenesis (wrong treatment and side-effects)

Constitution

'Constitution' is quite a broad term, and basically covers the overall level of health, resulting from a combination of inheritance, and the path that you have taken in your life up to the current point.

Problems inherited at birth, which we might call genetic, or which developed in childhood as a result of trauma, malnutrition, abuse, neglect, or inappropriate or unhelpful mental, emotional or spiritual influences, will naturally have a lasting effect and may colour the individual's health for the rest of their life.

In these cases, although it is impossible to go back in time and change the cause, it is quite possible to manage and mitigate the effects, and Chinese medicine can be extremely useful in many cases of 'constitutional' conditions.

Nutrition

Diet and nutrition has always been an important factor in health and well-being, although in early Chinese medicine malnutrition would probably have been the biggest concern, while now we have dietary problems of a very different kind. For more on the important role of nutrition in Chinese medicine, see Chapter 10.

Occupation

There are many and varied health problems that can be associated with work, both physical and mental/emotional.

Physical factors include poor posture and lack of exercise for office workers or those who spend a lot of time driving, excessive wear and tear and overwork of some physical workers, and extreme environments such as working in very cold, hot, or loud conditions.

Work can also be a cause of mental and emotional stress, dissatisfaction, boredom and frustration, which can have a considerable impact on health (see Internal Causes, above.)

While it not generally possible to simply give up work or move to a different job, these factors must be considered as potential causes of disease, and as with constitutional problems, Chinese medicine can often offer a number of ways to reduce or eliminate the negative effects on health.

Overwork

Overwork includes not only physical but also mental and emotional overwork. Put simply, if you overdo it in any area, you will exhaust your Qi and become Deficient. Over time, this will lead to illness. In my experience, it is mental and emotional 'overwork' that plagues so many people, which leads to frequent or enduring tiredness and exhaustion.

Sex and Relationships

Relationships with other people can be a source of great healing and support, and also a cause of stress and illness. Your interactions with those around you are interactions of your Qi with theirs, and every interaction will have its effect. Managing these relationships can be an important part of overall health and well-being.

Excessive sexual activity is also considered to be potentially harmful to health, especially for men. This is because Jing (Essence) is lost with ejaculation. What counts as 'excessive' depends on overall health and age, and naturally the whole subject is also tied up with societal and cultural values.

Trauma

Physical trauma includes all kinds of accident and injury, including burns, stings and so on.

Chinese medicine can be useful in these cases to speed and encourage healing, and to reduce or treat after-effects such as weakness, scarring, stiffness and so on.

Parasites and Poisons

Not much needs to be said about parasites and poisons, as they are such obvious disease causing factors. For serious cases of either, prompt treatment by Western medicine is recommended, and can of course be life saving.

Iatrogenesis

Iatrogenesis is the medical term given to illness or disease *caused* by medical treatment. It includes problems caused by incorrect treatment, and also side effects of treatment.

By its very nature, Chinese medicine rarely causes these kinds of problems, although it is possible, if treatment is carried out incorrectly. More commonly, Chinese medicine is used to counteract the side-effects of Western treatments. For instance, it is often used alongside chemotherapy treatment for cancer in order to strengthen the body and reduce side-effects.

Chinese medicine is also of great value in helping with the recovery from surgery.

CHAPTER 4

Using Chinese Medicine: 3 Steps To Radiant Health

When it comes to the practice of Chinese medicine, there are 3 steps that lead from illness, poor health and under-functioning, then to good health, and on to an optimum state of health and well-being. Only by following these steps can Chinese medicine be truly effective, and I always base my own clinic around this model. I call this process 'The 3 Steps To Radiant Health'.

Step 1: Diagnose Energetic Imbalance

This crucial first step makes use of detailed questioning along with ancient Chinese diagnostic tools such as pulse and tongue diagnosis, to develop an in-depth understanding of the current state of your Qi. This step identifies any problems or imbalances that may be affecting your health or quality of life.

This is an holistic (whole-person) process that takes into account all aspects of your health, life situation and constitution. It is an entirely different process to the diagnosis that you may receive if you go to your GP or another Western medical professional.

Step 2: Treat Current Conditions

Following on from the Chinese Diagnosis, the obvious next step is to treat any current conditions or health problems. This is only possible once step 1 has been thoroughly completed. During Step 2, the focus is on treatment of the main underlying imbalance(s) in order to alleviate troubling symptoms and restore quality of life.

Generally speaking, the longer you have had a particular problem, the longer it will take to treat. If you just put your back out yesterday digging the garden, one session of acupuncture or tui na might be all it takes to sort it out. However, if you've had migraines for the past 10 years, it will take a longer and more involved course of treatment.

For a more chronic (long-term) condition, or in complex cases, treatment should normally be quite frequent at the beginning – probably weekly, maybe even more often. Once you begin to see progress, you can usually start to space the sessions out further apart.

Step 3: Cultivate Radiant Health

Step 3 is when you move from treatment into maintenance and health-cultivation. This is the stage of 'nourishing life' (yang sheng).

Sometimes, it is not possible to completely 'cure' a condition, in which case this is a maintenance phase. A good example might be something like osteoarthritis, where there is a structural issue. In cases like this there is a bony growth, or some other problem with the physical structure of the body, which cannot be removed. During step 2 (treatment) the focus is on restoring movement, alleviating pain, and dealing with any other symptoms. Once the condition is under control, you move to step 3, and all that's needed are occasional maintenance 'top-ups'.

Step 3 is more than just maintenance though, it is also where the important and valuable work of health-cultivation and 'nourishing life' is carried out. This means that you continue to work on underlying energetic imbalances or weaknesses in order to strengthen and regulate the entire system. The effect is stronger immunity, more energy, less stress, more adaptability, greater reserves, and an easier, more relaxed engagement with life. This is radiant health!

During Step 3, sessions are normally something like once per month or every 6 weeks.

Section 2

Diagnosis

CHAPTER 5

Step 1 of 3: Diagnose Energetic Imbalance

To the uninitiated, the diagnostic system used by acupuncturists, Chinese herbalists and other practitioners of Chinese medicine can seem outlandish, outdated, and incomprehensible. But look a little deeper, and you find a remarkable framework for understanding the fundamental functions and dysfunctions of the human being. It is a deep and rich system that provides us with a unique insight into the nature of health and disease, and it's as useful and applicable in the modern world as it ever was in ancient China.

With talk of Qi, Yin, Yang, and other Chinese terms its language can sound arcane and unscientific, but these ancient terms reveal a penetrating insight into the human condition. Once we understand that this is a fundamentally different way of viewing health and illness we can start to apply the concepts of Chinese medicine to better understand ourselves and the world around us.

The complex diagnostic system used by Chinese medical practitioners underlies all of the different Chinese therapies, so an acupuncturist's diagnosis of a patient will be the same as a herbalist's – it is only the treatment that is different. This is what unites the 5 Branches of Chinese medicine, and because they 'speak the same language' it also means that they work very well together.

Because of the holistic nature of Chinese medicine, and the understanding of the interconnectedness of the many different systems that make up a human being, diagnosis is necessarily a 'whole-person' affair.

During the diagnosis stage of your treatment, your practitioner will be getting a feel for you as a whole, not only the disease or condition (if any) that you have gone for help with, but also the whole of your health and life. This is not a process of diagnosing a disease, as Western medicine does, but a process of understanding a person. In other words, although you may have the same 'condition' as someone else according to Western medicine, you are unique, your exact symptoms are unique, and so your diagnosis and treatment will also be unique to you.

Viewing the body, mind, emotions, spirit and environment as related systems, forming a web of interacting influences and exchanges, the Chinese medicine practitioner looks for the places where balance has been lost, and imbalance has set in. Rather than use disease labels such as 'migraine', 'depression' or 'sciatica', the Chinese Medicine practitioner looks for the underlying cause or causes of the symptoms based on the individual's own unique experiences. He or she is looking for a set of signs or indicators for one or more named imbalances, which we call 'Patterns Of Disharmony', or simply 'Patterns'.

Patterns are a combination of signs and symptoms that can be mental, emotional, physical or spiritual. They describe the underlying state of a persons energy, and thus their health and current symptoms, if any.

Because each person will have a different experience of health and illness, no two diagnoses are exactly the same. This means that there is no direct link between a 'disease' and a Pattern. For instance, migraines could be caused by a number of different Patterns, such as 'Phlegm', 'Full Heat' or 'Deficient Yin'. Similarly, Patterns can manifest in different ways, so someone with the Pattern of Yin Deficiency may complain of dry skin, anxiety or insomnia, among other things.

This means that similar diseases or conditions may have very different treatments, depending on the exact diagnosis. This is summed up in the saying 'one disease, many treatments, one treatment, many diseases'.

Diagnostic Theories

There are a great many different theories that can be brought to bear in the process of diagnosis, depending on the individual situation, and the practitioner's preferences, training and experience.

The '8 Principles' is one of the fundamental diagnostic theories - a simple way of distinguishing the basics of a condition on the basis of 4 sets of pairs: Yin/Yang, Hot/Cold, Internal/External and Deficient/Excessive. These are the terms that are mainly used in the descriptions of the main imbalances that follow in the next chapter. For instance, a condition may be characterised by too much heat in the body, in which case it would be Yang, Internal, Hot and Excessive.

Diagnosis can also be made by the climatic factors (Wind, Heat, Cold, Dampness and Dryness) or by the state of the substances (Qi, Blood, Body Fluids) or by the system of the 5-elements. Slightly more complex systems of diagnosis also exist, for instance the '6 classifications' is based on the channels or meridians, and describes, among other things, the stages and progression of an external condition such as a cold or flu.

This very brief dip into diagnostic theories should be enough to show that this is a highly skilled process, and also far too much to go into here! And in any case, there is no need for you to learn the entirety of Chinese diagnostic theory, that is your practitioner's job. That being said, the chapters that follow will introduce the basics, to better understand the language and thinking behind your treatment.

Diagnostic Techniques

Diagnosis of a Pattern of Disharmony is carried out by a practitioner using a number of tools. These are traditionally known as the '4 Examinations', which are Looking, Listening/Smelling, Asking and Touching,

Looking is the most obvious way that a physician can get information about the state of a person's health. Posture, complexion, movements and mannerisms can all form part of the 'looking' section of diagnosis, but the most important is the appearance of the tongue, which we will explore later.

Listening & Smelling are probably the least used clinically, but obviously coughing, wheezing or other sounds associated with the Lungs can be very useful. The tone or quality of the voice may also be revealing.

'Asking' will normally form the bulk of a physician's diagnosis, as you would expect. When you go to see a practitioner of Chinese medicine, don't be surprised if they ask you lots of questions that don't seem to have anything to do with your condition or complaint – remember that they are trying to get a broad picture of your overall state of health.

The last of the 4 Examinations is touching. This can include palpation of acupoints or parts of the body to see if there is any pain, swelling, hardness, heat or other interesting signs or symptoms. Touching also includes Pulse Diagnosis (see below)

Pulse Diagnosis:

The art of Chinese Pulse diagnosis is extremely complex, and takes many years and a great deal of practice to even learn the basics. However, it is a remarkable diagnostic tool that can reveal a lot about your health.

The pulse is taken on both wrists at the radial artery, using three fingers at a time, giving a total of 6 different pulse readings, each with a different significance.

When a trained practitioner takes the pulse, they are looking for differences between the feeling at each finger, as well as an overall sense of the 'quality' of the pulse, which can give very detailed information about the state of the person's Qi.

This may sound a bit strange, and you might find it hard to believe that there can be much difference between the pulse on one arm and the pulse on the other, let alone from one finger to the next on the same arm. But if you take a moment to feel your own pulse on both sides or, better still, try it on someone else, you will quickly begin to feel some variations.

The 6 different finger positions each correspond to a different organ in the body, for instance, one position reflects the state of the Lungs, and another the Heart. You will also notice your practitioner pressing with different amounts of force, this is to check variations of the pulse at different depths.

In my clinic, people are often amazed at the things that I can pick up on the pulse. I usually take the pulse at the end of the diagnosis, after a fair bit of discussion has already taken place. Sometimes the pulse reveals something that we have not already talked about, maybe an old or ongoing condition or symptom that my client has completely forgotten to mention – so when I ask them about it, it seems like magic!

There are 29 basic pulse qualities which a skilled pulse-reader can identify, each with a different diagnostic significance. These have unusual names that attempt to describe what the pulse feels like, but there is really no way that words can accurately describe the subtleties of the pulse qualities.

The 29 Pulse Qualities

Floating, Drumskin, Surging, Vacuous, Scallion Stalk, Scattered, Soft, Deep, Weak, Hidden, Confined, Slow, Moderate, Rapid, Racing, Replete, Bowstring, Tight, Long, Short, Stirring, Slippery, Choppy, Fine, Faint, Large, Bound, Regularly Interrupted and Skipping

Pulse diagnosis is one of the most difficult diagnostic skills to learn, and takes many years of practice - When you put together the 6 pulse positions, each taken at 3 depths, and the 29 pulse qualities you have a very complicated system!

Some examples:

A 'fine' or 'thin' pulse feels very narrow – more like a piece of thread than a piece of string. It indicates Deficiency, often of Blood.

A 'floating' pulse is felt strongly at the surface but disappears under pressure. It can have different meanings, but sometimes indicates that the Qi is at the surface of the body, in order to fight off an invasion such as a cold or flu.

A rapid pulse is simply faster than normal. It tends to indicate Heat in the system.

Tongue Diagnosis:

Alongside the pulses, tongue diagnosis is the other main tool used by all practitioners of Chinese medicine to help to discern the state of the Qi. Most people have never taken much notice of their tongue (let alone anyone else's!) and it can be surprising at first to see how much the tongue can change from day to day.

The main things that we look for in the tongue are the colour of the tongue body (i.e. the tongue itself), the shape and size of the tongue, the location and depth of any cracks, and the colour and thickness of the coating of the tongue, sometimes called the tongue moss or fur.

Just as the pulse is divided in 6 different positions, the tongue is also divided up into different areas, which correspond to different organs. For instance the tip of the tongue represents the Heart, so if the tip of the tongue is bright red, that indicates Heat in the Heart.

If the tongue is pale and/or thin, it normally indicates a Deficiency of some kind. If it is bright red, Heat, and if purple tinged, Stagnation. A swollen tongue with tooth marks down the edges normally points to a weakness in the digestive system and Dampness.

A yellow coating also shows Heat, and a thick, sticky looking tongue coating indicates Phlegm. Cracks point to a weakness in the organ that corresponds to the area of the tongue that the crack appears, and can also indicate Yin Deficiency.

Like the pulse diagnosis, putting these many signs together is no easy task, but once again this is a vital skill in the Chinese medicine practitioner's toolbox. The state of the tongue can really help to identify the state of the Qi, and is an essential part of diagnosis.

CHAPTER 6

The Main Disharmonies

THE PATTERNS OF DISHARMONY

The Chinese way of looking at health and wellness is all about balance and harmony, so it makes sense that illness and disease is described in terms of imbalance. It is when our system loses its balance that disease arises.

There is much that could be said about the nature of Qi, Blood, Yin, Yang and Body Fluids. The constant and dynamic interplay of these substances, the functioning of the organs, the influence of the environment, the role of emotions, and much more, all come together to make up the complex set of inter-related systems that are a human being.

But this is a book about the practice of medicine, which means the fixing, tuning and strengthening of these systems, and restoring balance. Hence, I will focus here on the *imbalance*, and how your diagnosis might look when you go to see a practitioner.

Imbalances, also called 'Patterns Of Disharmony', or simply 'Patterns' take many forms, but they fall into a few main categories, which I will describe here. They are called 'Patterns' because they consist of a number of symptoms from different systems which commonly occur together, and so form a distinct pattern. These symptoms may not be obviously related in Western scientific terms but they make sense when viewed from the point of view of Chinese medicine, and taking into account the connections between all the different systems in the body and mind.

For each Pattern I list some of the main symptoms that will normally go with that particular Pattern, but remember that diagnosis relies on a number of factors. You will probably never have all the associated signs and symptoms for any given Pattern – as a guide you could consider that if you have most of the signs and symptoms on the list, then you probably (but not necessarily) have that particular imbalance, to a certain degree.

The only way to be sure is to visit a qualified Chinese medicine practitioner - they will be able to ask the right questions, take your pulses, look at your tongue and use other diagnostic methods to work out exactly what's going on!

Some organs are particularly prone to certain kinds of imbalances, and these are also listed in the sections below. The different organs are described in more detail in the next chapter.

Qi Deficiency

'Qi' is the term for our basic energy and life-force. A deficiency of Qi means an under-functioning in some way. The general feeling is of being tired and run-down. We have all experienced Qi Deficiency when we feel tired having 'over done it', but this normally recovers quickly. Long term Qi Deficiency can often arise from burning the candle at both ends or suffering from long term stress.

Qi is made in the body from the food we consume and the air we breathe. A weakness in the digestive system or Lungs, or poor quality food or air can all contribute to Qi deficiency.

To remedy Qi deficiency, it is important to eat and sleep well, breathe deeply, and get enough rest and 'down time'. In terms of therapies, any of the branches of Chinese medicine can help this Pattern.

Symptoms:

- Low energy levels
- Weakened immunity
- Reduced appetite
- Shortness of breath or wheezing
- Sweating during the daytime, without exertion
- Poor digestions, and a tendency to loose stools
- A weak pulse

Organs Effected: Lung, Spleen, Heart, Kidney

Yang Deficiency (or 'Empty Cold')

Yang is the Hot energy of the body. When it is deficient we feel cold, low and tired. Yang deficiency (also called 'Empty Cold') is a progression of Qi deficiency, so it has all the symptoms of Qi deficiency, plus feelings and symptoms relating to coldness.

The feeling of Yang Deficiency is cold, tired and unmotivated. There is often fear and withdrawal from the world – an unwillingness or fear of engaging.

Yang deficiency is not a sudden, acute condition, it develops slowly over time. It is made worse by eating a heavy or rich diet, by cold foods and environments, and by having a sedentary lifestyle.

Yang Deficiency can also occur alongside Yin deficiency, which complicates the picture, and leads to a mixture of symptoms of Heat and Cold together.

To remedy Yang Deficiency try to keep warm all the time (especially round your kidney area) and avoid too much cold and raw food. Incorporate some warming spices into your diet, such as cinnamon, ginger and garlic. Movement, action and excitement are all yang qualities, so bringing these into your life any way you can will help to strengthen the Yang.

The gently warming treatment known as 'moxibustion' (normally carried out by acupuncturists) can greatly benefit Yang Deficient conditions. Nutritional therapy and herbs are also useful.

Symptoms - As for Qi Deficiency, Plus:

- Feeling Cold
- Cold hands and/or feet
- Pale face
- Not feeling thirsty, and preferring hot drinks
- Frequent pale coloured urination
- Low energy
- Lack of drive and motivation
- Low libido
- Needing lots of sleep
- Weak and slow pulse
- Pale tongue

Organs Effected: Spleen, Heart, Kidney

Blood Deficiency

The word 'Blood' as it is used in Chinese medicine has a much broader meaning than the word as it is normally used in English. Blood is the counterpart of Qi. It nourishes, moistens and grounds us.

Like Qi, Blood is formed out of the foods we eat, so Blood deficiency often accompanies digestive problems or poor diet. Blood deficiency is more common in women, and vegetarians.

When the Blood is Deficient you can feel weak, un-grounded and like you're not 'in' your own body. There is often a low level background anxiety.

To remedy Blood deficiency it is important to eat nutritious, easy to digest food. Iron containing foods such as red meat and green leafy vegetables are particularly good. Chronic Blood deficiency in vegetarians can be slow to sort out, and in these cases a detailed dietary analysis from a Chinese Nutritionist may be useful. Herbs can also help.

As this is a Deficiency Pattern, getting enough rest is also important to allow you to recharge. Moving and using the body (for instance in dance, sports or t'ai chi) will help you to feel more centred and grounded, so will physical touch, whether that's a hug or a massage.

Symptoms:

- Dull or sallow complexion
- Dry skin and/or hair, or hair loss
- Thin or emaciated body
- Dizziness on standing

- Blurred vision or 'floaters' in the visual field
- Pale lips
- Weak or brittle nails
- Poor memory
- General anxiety
- Scanty menstruation
- Cramp or muscle spasms
- Trouble dropping off to sleep
- A weak or thin pulse
- Thin and/or pale tongue

Organs Effected: Heart, Liver

Yin Deficiency (Or 'Empty Heat')

Yin has a cooling, moistening quality, and when deficient it can lead to feelings of heat and dryness. It is common in people who are always on the go and don't get enough rest. Menopausal symptoms such as hot flushes are often due to Yin Deficiency.

The feeling of Yin Deficiency is rushed, anxious, and ungrounded. In my clinic, people with this imbalance often describe feeling 'tired but wired'.

Yin deficiency can be caused or aggravated by too much stimulation (mental, emotional or physical.) Foods which have a Heating or stimulating effect will also make Yin Deficiency worse (see Chapter 10)

Yin Deficiency can also occur alongside Yang deficiency, which complicates the picture, and leads to a mixture of symptoms of Heat and Cold together.

To remedy Yin Deficiency it is important to get enough rest and quiet time, and to switch off the mind. Meditation, t'ai chi or yoga can help. Make sure to drink enough water, and avoid coffee (including decaf.) Relaxing 'yin style' tui na massage can also be very beneficial as a treatment for this Pattern.

Symptoms:

- Getting hot in the late afternoon or evening
- Hot flushes
- Night sweats
- Restless or interrupted sleep
- Vivid dreams

- Hot hands and feet
- Flushed cheeks
- Feeling restless
- Dry throat, especially at night
- A weak and rapid pulse
- Bright red tongue, with little coating or many cracks

Organs Effected: Lung, Heart, Kidney, Liver, Stomach.

Jing (Essence) Deficiency

Jing, sometimes translated as 'essence', is the deep, enduring life force. It is your reserve of energy, and governs your growth and maturity, and your ability to procreate. Jing deficiency can also be seen as a combination of Yin and Yang deficiency.

Jing deficiency in adults is a chronic condition that normally develops slowly over years, or can be inherited at birth. It can follow long periods of stress or illness. There is normally a weakness in overall functioning, with poor immunity, tiredness, sluggish digestion and other non-specific signs and symptoms. The feeling of Jing deficiency is of complete exhaustion, with nothing left in reserve.

Jing deficiency is slow to remedy. T'ai chi or chi kung practice can be beneficial. A good diet is essential. Deep rest and rejuvenation over a long period will replenish Jing – it is important not to keep 'overdoing it'. Treatment from a practitioner of Chinese Medicine is recommended.

Symptoms - infants and children:

- Late fontanelle closure
- Slow development
- Failure to thrive
- Brittle bones

Symptoms - adults:

- Brittle bones
- Poor teeth
- Poor memory
- Weak or sore lower back

- Premature senility
- Infertility
- Early greying or loss of hair
- No reserves of energy
- Unable to regulate temperature
- Weak pulse

Organs Effected: Kidney

Full Cold

Full Cold is the accumulation of too much Coldness in the system. This can be due to exposure to environmental cold, or eating too many foods with a Cold energy. Full Cold often co-exists with Empty Cold (Yang Deficiency) and the 2 are often treated the same.

To remedy Full Cold, follow the same guidelines as for Empty Cold - try to keep warm all the time (especially round your kidney area) and avoid too much cold and raw food. Incorporate some warming spices into your diet, such as cinnamon, ginger and garlic.

The warming treatment known as 'moxibustion' (normally carried out by acupuncturists) can greatly benefit this condition.

Symptoms:

- Feeling cold
- Cold hands and feet
- Desire for warm places
- Lack of thirst
- Lack of perspiration
- Abundant pale urination
- Blue tinge to tongue or face
- Slow but strong pulse
- Possible fixed, constricting pain

Organs Effected: Stomach, Lungs (as Wind-Cold)

Full Heat

Full Heat, sometimes also called 'Fire' is more intense and has stronger symptoms than Empty Heat. The Heat disturbs the body and mind, and a person with Full Heat will normally have a short fuse! It is often caused by long-term 'bottling' of emotions, or eating too many heating foods.

Full Heat can also effect specific parts of the body, for instance Heat in the joints may cause arthritis.

To remedy Full Heat cut out chilli, spices and coffee from the diet, and find a way to safely 'let of steam' or relax. Acupuncture, herbs or tui na are all effective treatments. T'ai chi or chi kung can be very useful, too.

Symptoms:

- Redness (e.g. red face and red eyes)
- Thirst
- Feeling very hot all over
- Scanty, dark coloured urination
- Constipation
- Rapid and strong pulse
- Easily angered / short tempered
- Migraines or headaches
- Red tongue with yellow coating
- Bleeding, e.g. nosebleeds

Organs Effected: Heart, Liver, Stomach, Lungs, Intestines

Qi Stagnation

In health the Qi flows in a smooth and uninterrupted way. The term 'Qi Stagnation' indicates that there is a disruption to the flow of Qi.

This is probably the most common Pattern, as the main causes of Qi Stagnation are stress and unexpressed or stifled emotions, which are pretty much a normal part of modern life!

Qi stagnation implies a blockage on some level, this could be mental, physical or emotional. Things do not flow as smoothly as they could. There are 'ups and downs', with stresses, pains or difficulties that come and go.

The feeling of Qi Stagnation is frustrated and blocked. It is the opposite of feeling free, calm and relaxed. The word 'should' describes a state where there is a feeling that something 'should' be done even though you don't want to do it – this is classic Qi Stagnation territory!

To remedy Qi Stagnation, try to reduce stress in any way you see fit. Take some exercise and stretch and move the body. Indulging your creative side, and expressing your thoughts and emotions also helps. Play, and have fun! Acupuncture and tui na massage are excellent therapies.

Symptoms:

- Pains that come and go, and are worse with stress
- Depression and/or irritability
- Pain or discomfort in the chest and/or ribs
- Mood swings

- Irritability or frustration
- Frequent sighing
- Muscle cramp
- Clumsy, uncoordinated or inelegant movement
- PMS

Organs Effected: Heart, Liver

Blood Stagnation / Stasis

Blood requires Qi to flow round the body, so Blood Stagnation (also called 'Blood Stasis') is always accompanied by a degree of Qi Stagnation. However, where Qi stagnation comes and goes, Blood Stagnation is fixed and enduring.

Blood Stagnation may manifest as fixed lumps and masses in the body – for instance fibroids, and some cancers.

To remedy Blood Stagnation you need to remedy Qi stagnation (see above) as well as using stronger treatments to move the Blood. Seek the advice of a qualified Chinese Medical Practitioner.

Symptoms:

- Fixed, stabbing pain
- Fixed abdominal lumps
- Purple lips, and/or purplish tinge to tongue
- Varicose veins or dark 'thread veins'
- Bleeding with dark blood
- Menstruation with dark blood, pain, and clots

Organs Effected: Heart

Dampness

Dampness underlies many diseases and health conditions, especially chronic and complex ones. Dampness is essentially pathological fluid, which causes swelling, weight gain, and difficulty shifting weight. All kinds of secretions imply dampness – for instance, weeping skin conditions and mucous. Dampness can also lodge in the joints, causing heaviness, stiffness and swelling.

The feeling of Dampness is heavy, slow, muddled and lethargic. It is as if a fog has seeped into the body and mind, weighing everything down and making concentration difficult. The 'brain-fog' typical of conditions such as fibromyalgia is normally due to Dampness.

Dampness combines with Heat to form Damp-Heat or with Cold to form Cold-Damp. In these cases, treatment is required for both the Dampness and the Heat or Cold.

Dampness relates to a weak digestive system, and can be hard to shift. Eating a good, easily digestible diet is essential, as well as avoiding dairy products, refined sugars and processed foods. Dampness has a heavy quality, and tends to settle, so movement helps to disperse it. All of the branches of Chinese Medicine make good treatments for Dampness, but Nutrition is key.

Symptoms:

- Heavy sensation in the body
- Mucous or bodily secretions
- Lack of appetite

- Congested or heavy feeling just below the chest
- Sticky taste in the mouth
- Muzzy head
- Symptoms worse upon waking, and with damp weather
- Oedema or water retention
- Trouble losing weight

Organs Effected: Spleen, Intestines. Damp-Heat can effect the Stomach, Liver, Gallbladder and Bladder.

Phlegm

Phlegm can be considered a development of Dampness. It takes two forms:

Substantial Phlegm: Mucous in the nasal passages, lungs etc. Like Dampness, Phlegm is often differentiated into Hot and Cold types:

Hot-Phlegm: Yellow and sticky phlegm, hard to expectorate, red face, dry mouth etc.
Cold-Phlegm: White watery phlegm, easy to expectorate, nausea, feeling of cold, pale face etc.

Insubstantial Phlegm: Can manifest as soft lumps internally or under the skin (e.g. some cysts or fibroids). Is also implicated in psychological disease, called 'Phlegm misting the Heart' and in many chronic muscle, bone or joint condition such as arthritis.

With any kind of phlegm the tongue has a thick 'sticky' coating.

Like dampness, phlegm can be hard to shift. Once it sets in, its sticky, heavy, cloying nature means it tends to hang around. Phlegm is a part of most chronic and complex conditions.

To treat Phlegm, nutrition is important. Exercise and movement can also be useful.

Organs Effected: Lungs, Spleen, Heart

Wind (External Invasions)

The term 'external invasion' in Chinese medicine describes anything that attacks the body from outside. Examples are colds, viruses, flu etc. This is also known as 'External Evils' or 'External Wind', but is not related to Internal Wind (see next page)

Wind normally comes and goes quickly. Any of the 5 branches of Chinese medicine can help either to fight off the invasion, or to strengthen immunity to stop you from succumbing in the first place.

Symptoms:

- Sudden onset
- Pain or discomfort that comes or goes, mainly in the upper body
- Dislike of wind and/or cold
- Runny nose
- Sneezing
- Chills and/or fever
- Body aches

Most common kinds of Wind:

Wind-Heat: More fever than chills, often with inflammation and sore throat
Wind-Cold: More chills than fever, often with aches, pains and stiffness

Organs Effected: Lung

INTERNAL WIND

Internal Wind relates to the Liver, and can have many causes. Just as wind in the environment causes things to move around, so Wind in the body also causes uncontrollable movements. Symptoms can be very varied, but the general manifestations include tremors or shaking, tics, numbness, dizziness, and in more severe cases, convulsions or paralysis.

Internal Wind can have a number of different causes, for instance extreme Heat in the body, Deficiency of Blood or a specific Pattern of Heat called 'Liver Yang Rising'. It is generally a complex and chronic problem, and further advice should be sought from a qualified practitioner.

Organs Effected: Liver

'Patterns' Case Study – Janet

Janet came to see me for help with her Irritable Bowel Syndrome (IBS). She was 39, and worked in an office in a job she found stressful. She was also very busy, and had 2 young children.

She had started suffering with IBS 3 or 4 years ago, during a particularly difficult and stressful time in her life. She had approached her GP who had referred her to a specialist. A number of tests showed no problems in her gut, and her blood tests came back normal. She was diagnosed with IBS and given a standard list of foods to avoid, which she found didn't really help at all.

Her symptoms were bloating, discomfort and cramps in the stomach area after eating, with alternating constipation and diarrhoea. Some foods seemed to particularly set her off more than others, and she had noticed that she was much worse when stressed.

Janet also suffered with PMS, especially mood swings and cramps. She also experienced muscle cramp in her calves at different points throughout the month. Her energy levels were very low.

Janet's pulse was weak overall, and also had a 'wiry' quality. Her tongue was pale and swollen with a thick coating and tooth marks down the side.

Diagnosis:

Janet's problems with digestion, tiredness, swollen tongue and weak pulse all point to Qi deficiency. The PMS, mood swings, cramp, wiry pulse quality, and the fact she is worse when stressed all show Qi stagnation.

For Janet, these are the 2 main imbalances, in broad terms. The second important part of diagnosis is to identify the particular organs that are effected, and it's that which I'd like to turn to in the next Chapter. We'll come back to Janet and flesh out her diagnosis some more later.

Chapter 7

The Organs

The Patterns described in the previous chapter indicate the overall nature of the imbalance in question, but to make a complete diagnosis we also need to understand which aspect or area of the person is affected - this is where the organs come in.

It is important to understand that Chinese medicine practitioners use the names of organs in a different way than they are normally used by a Western trained medical practitioner, or in everyday use.

To make this distinction in writing, the first letter of the organ is normally capitalised to indicate the Chinese meaning. For instance 'lungs' means the lungs as we normally understand them in the West, but 'Lungs' with a capital 'L' indicates the Chinese notion of the organ.

This difference is important to grasp, because the Chinese understanding of an organ goes beyond it's physical location and structure, and includes a variety of related functions, not just physical but also mental and emotional.

For instance the Chinese understanding of the Heart includes the muscle in the chest that pumps blood around the body, and ALSO the network of blood vessels, the emotion of joy, and the ability to think and speak clearly. Similarly, the Lungs are related to the skin, the immune system, and grief, as well as the obvious function of breathing.

The list of possible correspondences for each organ is very long, and includes items such as flavour, colour, direction, season, time of day, sound and much more. These correspondences are often used diagnostically, and sometimes therapeutically. For instance, the colour associated with an organ can show as a hue to the skin on a certain part of the body, which has diagnostic use. The flavour association can also be relevant diagnostically, for instance if a particular flavour is craved, or strongly disliked, then that can sometimes indicate an imbalance in that organ. The flavours also have therapeutic use (see Chapter 10).

The organ that causes particular trouble is the Spleen, which in Chinese medicine is the main organ of digestion (in Western medicine the spleen has little to do with digestion). This is largely a translation problem – just remember that whenever you read or hear 'Spleen' in relation to Chinese medicine, that you should think 'digestive system'.

Organ Imbalances

There are 12 main organs, divided into 6 pairs. Each pair consists of a Yin and a Yang organ. The Yin organs are normally considered the more important than the Yang organs in terms of diagnosis, so it is the Yin organs which are described in detail below.

Not every kind of imbalance applies to every organ - The organs have different relationships with the substances (Qi, Blood, Yin, Yang etc.) and so each organ is prone to particular types of imbalance. For instance, the Liver is prone to Heat, so there are Patterns of 'Liver Fire' and 'Liver Yin Deficiency' but there is no 'Liver Cold' or 'Liver Yang Deficiency'.

In the descriptions that follow, a table at the beginning of the section for each organ describes the paired 'Yang' organ, and associated emotions, tastes and colours along with related body parts and main imbalances. Please note that this is not necessarily a full list of all possible imbalances for that organ, simply the most commonly encountered.

I have also given the elemental association for that organ, using the 5-element system. Some practitioners, particularly of 5-element acupuncture, prefer to talk in these terms. For instance an 'Earth imbalance' refers to the organs that are associated with the Earth element, which are the Spleen and Stomach.

'Suggested' Conditions

It is very important to remember that there is no direct 1-to-1 link between any Chinese imbalance, as diagnosed by your practitioner, and a Western disease label. All signs and symptoms must be taken as part of the bigger picture.

So, the suggestions that follow for kinds of illness and conditions that might come about to do with different organs are for illustrative purposes only, and there are almost always other interpretations. For instance, you will read that the Liver energy 'flares upwards' and can cause headaches. This does NOT mean that ALL headaches are caused by a Liver imbalance. The same goes for all other conditions or symptoms mentioned here.

Lungs

Yin Organ	Lungs
Yang Organ	Large Intestine
Element	Metal
Emotion	Grief, Sadness
Body Parts	Nose, Skin
Taste	Pungent
Colour	White
Main Imbalances	Qi Deficiency, Yin Deficiency, Phlegm, External Invasions

Breathing and Qi

Needless to say, the Lungs govern breathing, and all kinds of asthma, coughing, wheezing or other breathing problems involve the Lungs. When the Lungs are strong, breathing is deep, free and easy.

The Qi that you extract from the air is one of the two main components that you make your own personal Qi out of (along with the Qi from food) – therefore strong Lungs are essential for strong Qi.

The 'Tender Organ' and External Invasions

The Lungs are known as the 'tender organ'. They are in direct contact with the external world through the process of breathing, and also govern the skin and pores, which form the physical barrier to the world at large.

This makes the Lungs liable to 'attack' from external influences. The concept of 'External Evil' or 'Wind' attacking the Lungs corresponds to all kinds of colds, flu and viruses (see page 68)

Personal Boundaries

The Lungs are not only a boundary between interior and exterior physically, they also relate to mental and emotional boundaries. The Lung energy helps you to maintain your personal boundaries, and to make good decisions about what to let in and what to keep out.

A weakness or disruption to this function can result in boundaries that are too firm and strict, so that nourishment doesn't get in, or a lack of discernment so that not enough is kept out, and damaging and unhelpful influences are allowed in. This relates to self-esteem and self-respect, which are both strong in people with a strong Lung energy.

Nose, Throat and Voice

The Lungs govern the whole of the respiratory tract, including the nose and throat. When Lung Qi is strong, the nose and sinuses are clear and unblocked and you have a strong sense of smell.

A strong, clear voice also reflects strong Lungs, while a quiet, cracked or weak voice or finding that you 'lose your breath' or that your voice tires easily may indicate Lung deficiency.

Grief and Sadness

The Lungs are effected by Grief and Sadness, and a Lung weakness can make you more prone to these feelings. Like all emotions, grief is a natural response to loss, and is not pathogenic in itself, but it becomes a problem if it is repressed or hidden away.

In my experience extreme grief or sadness, or not being able to express grief, can seriously effect the Lungs, and this often manifests in the skin, which the Lung governs – this can come out in the form of a rash, eczema or similar condition.

Strengthening The Lung

To strengthen the Lung energy, practice deep and mindful breathing techniques to use the Lungs to their full capacity. A good upright posture to keep the Lungs open is important. Using the voice and breath in singing or public speaking can also be helpful.

Spleen

Yin Organ	Spleen
Yang Organ	Stomach
Element	Earth
Emotion	Worry, Over-thinking
Body Parts	Mouth, Muscles
Taste	Sweet
Colour	Yellow
Main Imbalances	Qi Deficiency, Yang Deficiency, Dampness, Phlegm

Spleen = Digestion!

Remember that when you see 'Spleen' in relation to Chinese Medicine it really means 'Digestive System' – so the Spleen is responsible for all aspects of digestion. Conditions such as constipation, diarrhoea, bloating after eating, food intolerance and indigestion will all involve the Spleen in some way.

Responsible for Qi and Blood

The Spleen is crucial for the production of Qi and Blood. It is the Spleen's job to extract the Qi from foods, and begin the process of converting it into Qi and Blood. This is why a strong digestive system and a good diet are essential for overall health.

The Spleen is said to govern the muscles, in the sense that if Qi and Blood are weak due to a Spleen deficiency the muscles become undernourished, and may become weak.

When there is a weakness of either Qi or Blood, the Spleen must be addressed.

Fluid, Dampness and Phlegm

The Spleen also has an important role in the fluid-metabolism of the body, as it receives the fluids from food and drink, processes them, and then transports them to other parts of the body. When this function is weak, fluid stagnates and congeals, becoming pathogenic Dampness or Phlegm.

The Spleen Is The Centre

The digestive organs are located in the centre of body, and are also at the centre of our energetic system. In all aspects of health and disease it is always vital to 'protect the centre' which means to avoid any kind of damage to the Spleen and Stomach. In this way, you keep the foundation of Qi and Blood strong, and prevent Dampness and Phlegm. This is why diet is such an important part of overall health and well-being.

The Spleen, Intellect and Worrying

The Spleen is also responsible for rational, logical thought, and a weakness in the Spleen can result in difficulties in this area. Similarly, over-thinking and worrying can damage the Spleen. This relationship between digestion and the mind is expressed in the English language in phrases such as 'food for thought', and it also explains why students often suffer with diarrhoea and other digestive problems, due to overuse of the intellect and subsequent weakening of the Spleen Qi.

Holding The Organs And Blood

The Spleen is said to have a lifting, supporting and holding function. It is responsible for 'holding' the muscles and organs in position, and when the Spleen is weak there can be sagging, drooping or even organ prolapse.

The Spleen also 'holds' the Blood in the vessels, so bleeding can sometimes be an indication of a problem with the Spleen.

Nourishment, Support And Caring

The Spleen is to do with nourishment on all levels. As well as receiving nourishment directly from food, a healthy Spleen also needs to receive emotional and spiritual nourishment. The Spleen energy responds to being held, touched, and cared for.

The ability to both give and receive support, and to care for others as well as allow yourself to be cared for, relies on a strong and healthy Spleen Qi. When the Spleen is strong, you can feel safe, secure, grounded and nourished.

Strengthening The Spleen

The Spleen responds to touching and being touched, whether that's a massage or a loving hug. Structure and safety are important, and so a good sense of 'home' is important.

Anything that you can do that feels nourishing will strengthen the Spleen, including (but not limited to) a good, natural and wholesome diet.

Heart

Yin Organ	Heart
Yang Organ	Small Intestine
Element	Fire
Emotion	Joy, Happiness
Body Parts	Eyes, Tongue
Taste	Bitter
Colour	Red
Main Imbalances	Qi Deficiency, Yang Deficiency, Blood Deficiency, Yin Deficiency, Qi Stagnation, Blood Stagnation, Phlegm, Full Heat

The Heart, Shen, And The Mind

The Heart houses the Shen ('spirit' or 'mind') and when the Heart is strong and its Qi is regulated, the mind is clear and sharp. When the Heart is weak or the Qi flow is stagnant there can be difficulties relating with others, agitation, insomnia, confused thinking and in extreme cases, hallucinations or distortions of reality. For this reason Heart imbalances are often involved in all kinds of mental health conditions and insomnia.

When the Shen is strong and unobstructed, there are feelings of joy and tranquillity. The Chinese character for the word 'Shen' depicts an empty vessel, which points to the nature of Shen, and the way to work with it. This 'emptiness' of the spirit refers to an absence of distractions, ties and complications – It is a state where the ego steps out of the way, where desires and fears dissolve and you experience a state of ecstatic peace and joy, in connection and unity with the infinite.

When the Heart is healthy, you are able to feel and experience a wide range of emotions, without any of them taking over, and you can easily make healthy connections with those around you.

The state of the Shen is reflected in the eyes, which are dull or glassy when the Shen is weak, and sparkly and alive when the Shen is strong.

The Emperor, and Emotions

Traditionally, the different organs were likened to different positions in the imperial court, to help to explain their functions. The Heart was given the highest possible role - Emperor.

This illustrates the importance of the Heart as the vessel of the Spirit, the highest aspect of ourselves, and also shows us the important role of emotions in health and illness, which is summed up in the saying 'all disease begins with the Heart'.

Although each organ has an associated emotion, the Heart houses the Shen which encompasses all of our emotional life, and all emotional problems will effect the Heart. Because all aspects of Qi are inter-related, emotional upsets can easily become physical conditions, and emotional disturbance is implicated in many illnesses.

Joy

The emotion particularly associated with the Heart is Joy, and a symptom of Heart imbalances is either a lack or an excess of Joy – in this case 'excessive joy' means manic or unnatural joy, and is often seen in people who laugh inappropriately for no reason.

Blood, The Cardiovascular System, And The Chest

Needless to say, the Heart governs the circulation of Blood around the body, including the whole of the cardiovascular system. The Heart is also involved in the production of Blood

On a physical level, pain and discomfort in the chest, palpitations, angina and heart disease are all related to the Heart.

Strengthening The Heart

To strengthen the Heart, you must work to develop and maintain relationships with others. You must also consider your relationship with and connection to your Higher Self, or to God, the Tao or whatever you believe in. All forms of spirituality and religion work with the Shen. Meditation and self-reflection are important.

Self-expression is also a way of freeing and strengthening Heart energy.

Kidneys

Yin Organ	Kidneys
Yang Organ	Bladder
Element	Water
Emotion	Fear, Shock
Body Parts	Ears, Knees, Lower Back
Taste	Salty
Colour	Black, Dark Blue
Main Imbalances	Qi Deficiency, Yin Deficiency, Yang Deficiency, Jing Deficiency

Jing, Yin And Yang

The Kidneys store the Jing, and are the source of all the Yin and Yang in the body. They are the foundation of life and the root of our physical bodies.

Jing is the life-force that you inherit from your parents, and which you gradually use up throughout your life. Its gradual decline over time accounts for balding, loss of hearing, failing eyesight and the other common signs of ageing.

Keeping the Kidney Jing strong is essential in order to maintain good health and vitality into old age, and maintaining high Jing levels is one of the key aims of many of the yang sheng self-cultivation practices (see Chapter 15) In fact, the Kidneys are unique among the organs because they have only deficiency Patterns, and no Patterns to do with excess – this is because you can't have too much Jing!

Strong and balanced Yin, Yang and Jing are essential for conception, so treating the Kidneys is important when there is infertility or difficulties conceiving. The balance of Yin and Yang also finds expression in our sexuality, and sexual problems can often relate to the Kidneys.

As the source of Yin and Yang of the body, a deficiency of Kidney Yin or Kidney Yang can easily effect other organs if it goes on for long enough. Similarly, a Yin or Yang deficiency of any organ will eventually effect the Kidneys as the deficient organ makes excessive demands for more Yin or Yang from the store held by the Kidneys. For this reason, the Kidneys are normally involved in any treatment for either Yin or Yang Deficiencies.

Hormones And The Kidneys

It is too simple to say that all hormonal problems relate to the Kidneys, but there is often some kind of Kidney disharmony involved when hormones are out of balance. This is largely due to the Kidney's relationship with the adrenal glands (which sit directly on top of the kidneys) – sometimes the Chinese word for the Kidneys is translated as 'Kidney-Adrenals' for this reason, although there is no concept of hormones or adrenal glands in Chinese medicine. That being said, the Western concept of adrenal fatigue is very close to Qi and Jing Deficiency in Chinese medicine.

Bones, Teeth, Back, And Knees

The Kidneys control the skeleton, and when the Kidneys are strong, the bones are strong. Weak or brittle bones or joints, arthritis and osteoporosis often involve the Kidneys.

The Kidneys also govern the lower back and the knees, and Kidney imbalances often show with weakness, pain or stiffness of these areas.

Dental problems may also involve the Kidneys due to their influence on the teeth.

Fear, Willpower and Memory

The strength of the Kidneys influences the strength of the mind in many ways. When Kidney energy is strong the mind is clear and strong. Weakness in the Kidneys can lead to muzzy or slow thinking and especially poor memory.

The strong, deep and enduring energy of the Kidneys is responsible for your Willpower, courage, sense of purpose, and the ability to see things through. It shows itself in the survival instinct - your will to live. When this strength is lacking, fear is the result.

Fluid Metabolism And Urination

Along with their paired organ the Bladder, the Kidneys play a key role in fluid metabolism in the body, and with urination. Conditions of the urinary system normally involve the Kidneys and/or Bladder.

Strengthening The Kidneys

To strengthen the Kidneys, make sure you have enough rest and downtime to recharge your stocks of Jing. Confront and deal with your fears, and engage fully with life. Eating a natural, wide ranging and wholesome diet is also important.

Pericardium And San Jiao

Yin Organ	Pericardium
Yang Organ	San Jiao
Element	Fire
Emotion	Joy
Body Parts	NA
Taste	Bitter
Colour	Red
Main Imbalances	NA

The Unusual Organs!

The Pericardium and the San Jiao are the 2 organs that cause the most confusion in Chinese Medicine. The Pericardium or 'Heart Protector' has functions that overlap with those of the Heart and the San Jiao, also known as the 'Triple Heater' or 'Triple Burner' is mainly used as a term to describe the 3 divisions of the body.

The Pericardium can be seen as an 'intermediary' between the Heart and the world outside, hence the name 'Heart Protector'. In practice though, the Pericardium is of less importance than the 5 other main organs (Lungs, Spleen, Heart, Kidneys and Liver) and individual Pericardium imbalances, although theoretically possible, are rarely diagnosed.

The San Jiao is called the organ 'with function, but no form' – it has no physical form of itself, and is best considered as a group of functions that belong to no particular organ. It is also known (misleadingly) as the 'Triple Heater' or 'Triple Warmer'.

The San Jiao includes the concept of three divisions in the body – The Upper Jiao is everything from the diaphragm upwards and contains the Lungs and Heart, the Middle Jiao is between the diaphragm and navel and contains the Stomach and Spleen, and the Lower Jiao is everything from the navel down, and contains the Kidneys and Bladder, Liver, Gall-Bladder and Intestines.

This way of talking is common among Chinese practitioners, as it provides a handy shorthand. For instance, you may hear talk of 'Qi Deficiency in the Upper Jiao' or 'Damp Heat in the Lower Jiao'.

San Jiao as a Transportation network

The San Jiao also acts as a transportation network, governing the formation and transportation of fluid around the body – a kind of system of waterways that irrigate the body. Disruption to this function could lead to symptoms of oedema or difficult urination, for instance.

Not A Thermostat!

I said that the name 'Triple Heater' is misleading, as some Western practitioners consider the San Jiao to be a kind of bodily thermostat, regulating temperature. This idea is foreign to traditional Chinese medicine. Body temperature is more to do with the balance of Yin and Yang, which is governed by the Kidneys.

Use In Acupuncture And Tui Na

Although diagnoses of these organs is uncommon, the Pericardium and San Jiao channels, and the points along them, are often used in acupuncture and tui na. As always with point selection, this will be on the basis of the location and functions of the individual points, which are used as and when needed. As both channels run along the arms, Pericardium and San Jiao points can be used for various conditions of the hand, wrist and arm, as well as for the specific internal effects of the different points.

Liver

Yin Organ	Liver
Yang Organ	Gallbladder
Element	Wood
Emotion	Anger
Body Parts	Eyes, Tendons & Ligaments
Taste	Sour
Colour	Green
Main Imbalances	Qi Stagnation, Blood Deficiency, Yin Deficiency, Full Heat, Damp-Heat, Internal Wind

Cycles And Free Flow

The Liver is all about the 'free flow' of Qi and Blood, and is intimately involved with all the cycles and fluctuations of the body from day to day and month to month.

When you have smooth, free flowing Qi you feel free, easy and unobstructed. When Qi flow is blocked or stagnant it causes pain and discomfort, mood swings and irritability. Stagnant Qi is erratic and volatile.

This free-flowing function of the Liver is easily disrupted by frustration or emotional repression, and as these are pretty much a part of modern life, Liver Patterns are extremely common! In my clinic, I find that Liver Qi Stagnation is one of the most common of all the imbalances.

The Liver is also closely involved with the Blood, and for women, the Liver is vital for a regular and symptom-free menstrual cycle. PMS, period pain and infrequent or irregular periods normally involve the Liver.

The Liver is easily effected by Heat, which manifests with symptoms such as anger, headache, red or irritated eyes, and high blood pressure.

The Liver and Creativity

Creation and expression are manifestations of a healthy and strong Liver energy. Like most things in Chinese medicine this is a two way process, so following creative pursuits is a good way of working with the Liver, and helping it to circulate Qi.

Regulates Muscular Tension, and effects the Head and Eyes

Part of the Liver's role is to regulate the state of tension or relaxation of the muscles. When the Liver is not functioning well, there can be muscle cramp or chronic tension.

The Liver is paired with the Gall-Bladder, and the Gall-Bladder channel runs all around the head, down the neck and along the tops of the shoulders. The nature of the Liver is to flare upwards, hence, Liver disharmonies often effect the head, neck and shoulders, in the regions of the gall-Bladder channel. For this reason, many kinds of headaches, migraine, and neck and shoulder tension involve the Liver.

The Liver is closely related to the eyes, and eye dryness, soreness, glaucoma , blurred vision or other eye problems can often have some involvement from the Liver.

The Liver and Wind

The Liver of all the organs is uniquely effected by Internal Wind, which describes an extreme lack of free-flow of Qi. Wind disrupts the smooth circulation of Qi, and causes ticks, tremors, fits and shaking.

The Liver And The Genitals

The Liver channel runs through the genitals for both men and women, and Liver disharmonies can cause problems to do with the genitals and sexual arousal (along with the Kidneys.)

Strengthening The Liver

The liver is 'softened' and 'relaxed' by creativity and movement. Stretching, dancing, and all co-ordinated or rhythmical movement will help. T'ai Chi and Qi Gong practice are very useful. Avoiding stress, and finding ways to safely express difficult emotions is very important.

Organs Case Study: Janet Revisited

Do you remember Janet, the IBS sufferer? So far we have identified Qi Deficiency and Qi Stagnation as her main Patterns. Now that you know a little about the organs you can give these two broad Patterns a home.

By the way, this is not the way that diagnosis is done in practice. The identification of the organs involved happens alongside the identification of the type of imbalance, but I've broken this fluid process into two for the purposes of this case study to make it easier to understand.

Janet's digestive problems clearly point to an under-functioning Spleen, so she has Spleen Qi Deficiency. And we know that it is the Liver that accounts for the smooth flow of Qi around the body. Her Qi Stagnation symptoms such a cramps, mood swings and PMS all relate to Liver function, so her second Pattern is Liver Qi Stagnation.

This particular set of 2 Patterns – Spleen Qi Deficiency and Liver Qi Stagnation - are so commonly found together that the pair is given its own name. When they occur together they are called 'Liver Invading Spleen' (there are also a few other combinations of Patterns given a separate name, but not many)

'Liver Invading Spleen' is a very common diagnosis for sufferers of IBS and other digestive problems, but it is worth pointing out again here that the Chinese diagnosis ALWAYS depends on the individual presentation. A different person with IBS may have a quite different Chinese diagnosis, and hence, a quite different treatment.

Mixed Patterns

Janet's case, described above, is typical but somewhat simplified. Most people in Western cultures who are suffering from chronic conditions have a mixture of Patterns, often many at a time, involving more than one organ. There may be 3, 4 or even more Patterns going on at once, each influencing the others – this is called a 'knotty condition' in Chinese medicine!

To treat knotty conditions requires sophisticated diagnostic skills and experience, and dedication on behalf of both the physician and the patient. As all the Patterns influence each other, a treatment that attempts to isolate and treat only one Pattern is rarely effective, and it can be helpful to address most or all of the relevant Patterns at once.

As treatment progresses, it is like slowly unpicking and untangling the 'knot' of signs, symptoms, causes and influences. Gradually things become clearer and less muddled, and the treatment plan continually and gradually adapts each time some new piece of information is unearthed, or a new connection discovered.

In my experience the best results for knotty conditions are obtained by using a combination of therapeutic approaches (i.e. more than one of the 5 branches of Chinese medicine)

This holistic, integrated approach can often reap benefits in complex cases when single treatments fail. The most skilled Chinese medicine practitioners are flexible enough to use appropriate treatments in combination, just as the ancient Chinese did, in response to the individual before them at the time. No two treatment plans are the same!

My hope is that this book can help you to understand the

wonderful world of Chinese medicine, and in doing so help you to understand your own health and well-being, but if you are ill, self-diagnosis and treatment is never recommended.

The more complex or 'knotty' the situation, the more important it is to seek professional advice. And needless to say, you should always seek advice from a qualified medical practitioner if you have any health conditions that concern you.

Section 3

Treatment

Chapter 8

Step 2 of 3: Treat Current Conditions

THE 5 BRANCHES OF CHINESE MEDICINE

Once diagnosis is complete, it is time to move onto step 2 of the 3 Steps To Radiant Health, and treatment can begin. There are traditionally said to be 5 branches of Chinese medicine, namely:

- Acupuncture
- Tui Na Massage
- Nutrition
- Herbalism
- T'ai Chi and Qi Gong

I will explore these in detail in the next few chapters.

These 5 Branches can be used singularly or combined together. There are times when one particular form of treatment is preferred, but in my experience an integrated approach to treatment that draws on 2 or more of these 5 branches often gives better, and faster results, especially for complex conditions.

That being said, sometimes it is quite suitable to use just one kind of therapy, depending on your needs and preferences. If you have a particular interest in a certain kind of therapeutic approach, or on the other hand if there's something that you don't like the sound of, then of course it makes sense to follow those inclinations.

Choosing A Practitioner

A good practitioner of Chinese medicine can sometimes become more than just a clinician. If you choose well, you may find someone who can be a guide, friend, and mentor. A life-long partner in your own journey towards optimum health and well-being, and someone who you can develop a real relationship with, who can get to know you, and who you may turn to for many different kinds of help at many different times in your life.

But How To Choose?

Firstly, it is very important that you get on well with your practitioner. You must have some kind of alignment of views, some understanding between you. If you don't have this connection then however skilled or qualified they are, you will never get the best out of them.

Your practitioner will want to talk to you about all aspects of your health, so it is important that you feel relaxed, and able to be open and honest, and share your thoughts and feelings. A good practitioner will go at your speed, not putting undue pressure on you, and will work WITH you, not ON you!

Obviously, length of time practising is a useful thing to consider, but may not be the most important factor. Someone who has been practising for 40 years will have more experience and skill than a new graduate, but I have met some highly talented and skilled Chinese medicine graduates, and some 'old-timers' who barely practice any more, have lost their enthusiasm, and are stuck in a rut.

If you have a specific condition that you are looking for help with, then somebody with experience treating that condition is obviously a bonus. But bear in mind that in Chinese medicine there is no clear one-to-one link between a Western diagnosed condition and a Chinese treatment – and the Chinese diagnostic system should allow any practitioner to diagnose and treat you, regardless of the Western disease label you have been given.

You may also want to look at professional memberships. Most Chinese medicine practitioners will belong to one or two organisations that act as a kind of 'governing body' for the profession. Here in the UK, there are a number of such bodies, with no one centrally held list, and no legal requirement to register with any particular group or organisation (the situation varies in other countries). This means that there is not much to choose between the different groups and memberships.

The best thing you can do is go on a personal recommendation if you can get one, if not, I recommend phoning a few local practitioners and asking them lots of questions. You might want to ask about their training and experience, what their particular approach to treatment is, if any, and which kinds of therapy or treatment they offer. They should be happy to talk to you about all of this kind of information – if not, put down the phone and try someone else!

As I have no doubt made clear, I firmly believe in an integrated approach to Chinese medicine – a classical, flexible way of working that can make use of any of the different therapeutic interventions, either alone or in combination, as the situation dictates.

In my clinic, I often have people come to me who already know what kind of treatment they want, maybe because they have had success with it before. Others come simply with a problem, condition or area of their life that they would like help with, but have no particular idea what kind of therapy they want. In any case, I will work with them to come to a suitable treatment plan, depending on their needs and wants at that particular time.

If this appeals to you, look for a practitioner who works this way – they may well use the label 'Classical Chinese Medicine' in their literature or on their website.

If you would like to find out more about my practice, you can do so at my website:

www.qi-therapies.com

Chapter 9

Acupuncture & Tui Na – The Channels & Acupoints

The Energetic Body

Most people are familiar with acupuncture, which involves the use of tiny needles at specific points in the body, in order to treat illness and maintain health. However, most have never heard of tui na, the Chinese massage and acupressure therapy. The crossover between the two is that they both work very directly with the 'energetic body' - the channels and acupoints.

According to this ancient understanding, our Qi flows around the body in a set pattern, following certain channels, sometimes called 'meridians'. These channels flow all around the body, creating a matrix of interconnecting pathways both on the surface, and within. They link and unify all parts of the body, carrying Qi and Blood, and connecting the interior and exterior.

The Channels

There are 12 standard channels, and 8 'extra' channels (also called vessels.) The 12 standard channels are each named after one of the internal organs, with which they connect (see box) There are also numerous smaller 'luo' channels which connect the main channels to each other, and to other parts of the body.

Organ Channels:	Extra Channels:
Lung	Ren (Conception Vessel)
Large Intestine	Du (Governing Vessel)
Stomach	Yin Heel Vessel
Spleen	Yang Heel Vessel
Heart	Yin Connecting Vessel
Small Intestine	Yang Connecting Vessel
Bladder	Girdle / Belt Vessel
Kidneys	Penetrating Vessel
Pericardium	
San Jiao	
Gall Bladder	
Liver	

The extra channels, or vessels, perform a number of functions, one of which is as a kind of 'overflow' for the organ channels. They also come into play in t'ai chi and chi kung practice.

Acupuncturists and tui na therapists mainly work with the 12 standard channels and the two extra channels which have their own acupoints – the Ren and Du (the other extra channels may share points where they overlap with the organ channels, but have none of their own)

Arranged along the channels are specific points, called 'acupoints' at which the Qi flow can be influenced. They are the 'gates' or 'valves' that an acupuncturist or tui na practitioner can use to access the flow of Qi and Blood around the body.

Traditional Chinese acupuncture recognises something like 400 acupoints, spread out all over the body. These points each have a Chinese name, and are also numbered along the channel. For instance the 36th point along the Stomach channel is just below the knee, it's number is Stomach-36 (abbreviated to 'St36') and it's name is *Zu San Li*.

The channel system helps to explain the actions of some of the acupoints. For example, St36, located on the leg, regulates and strengthens the digestive system. This makes little sense if you look at its physical location, but is quite understandable if you know that it is a point of the Stomach channel, which connects internally with the Stomach.

Another example is Kidney1 the 'bubbling spring', the only channel point on the sole of the foot. As the lowest point on the whole body, it helps to descend Qi from the head, and can be used for headaches, insomnia or over-thinking.

There are also a number of 'extra' points that are not located on, and are not related to, any particular channel. These tend to have quite specific functions, for instance the point 'anmian' located behind the ear, helps insomnia.

Finally, the category of points called 'ashi' points have no fixed location, and are determined by the practitioner by palpation.

The ashi point is simply a point of local tenderness or pain, and can sometimes (but not always) correspond with the Western concept of a 'trigger point'.

Which points are used?

An acupuncture or tui na practitioner will chose a set of points that will work together to restore balance and harmony to your system, based on the disharmony identified in the initial diagnosis. These could be located anywhere on the body, but generally speaking points will be taken from 3 different categories:

1. Local points
Points at or very near the problem area, if there *is* a specific area. For instance, for knee pain, a few points around the knee will probably be chosen.

2. Distal points
Points not at the problem area, but related to it via channel connections. The channels in the leg, for example, run up and down rather than across (this is generally true of the channels all over the body) so for knee pain, a distal point might be selected on the foot, choosing a point on the channel which connect to the area of pain at the knee.

3. Causal points
Points which deal with the root of the imbalance. So, if the pain in your knee is down to Dampness in the joint, a point to clear Dampness would be chosen. This could be anywhere on the body, depending on the specific action required.

ACUPUNCTURE

Acupuncture involves small needles, which are inserted into the body at the acupoints, in order to stimulate the effect of the point, and restore balance and harmony. Originally, thin slivers of stone or bamboo were used. As it wouldn't have been possible to make these too thin, the experience of acupuncture in those days was probably quite painful! These days acupuncturists use extremely thin stainless steel needles, typically around 0.2mm. They may range from 1cm to around 10cm in length, but 3-6cm long needles are normally used by most acupuncturists.

These days almost all acupuncturists use disposable needles, because of their ease of use and safety. The needles come in sterile packs, and are only used once, and then disposed of. Previously, metal needles were sterilised using an autoclave, but this practice has mainly died out and most of the professional bodies governing acupuncture practice in the West insist on disposable needles for their members.

Any number of needles may be used, depending on the practitioner, the style of acupuncture being practised, and the nature of the condition being treated. Normally something like 8-14 needles are used in one session.

Once the needles are inserted, they are moved gently to the correct depth, and then usually manipulated by the acupuncturist in order to make sure that the acupoint is active, and the treatment is having the desired effect. The depth of an acupoint is determined partly by which part of the body it is on, and partly by body shape and size. Generally speaking, on bigger or more fleshy parts of the body, the points are deeper.

A number of different manipulation techniques may be used to stimulate the point - for instance, the needle may be lifted up and down, or rotated between finger and thumb. The aim is to produce a sensation known as 'deqi', which is normally experienced as a dull, heavy feeling, but can also be felt as a tingling, fizzing or even itching. Once 'deqi' is felt, the point is said to be activated.

Different Styles Of Acupuncture

The main difference in styles of acupuncture is between the modern, Western ways of working (so called 'medical acupuncture') and the ancient, oriental styles ('traditional acupuncture'.) These two are so different, that to call them both by the name 'acupuncture' is quite misleading.

Medical Acupuncture is a recent creation, based entirely on the principles of Western scientific medicine. Training courses for qualified Western practitioners (such as GPs, nurses, physios etc.) are very short – typically around five days (or less!). This therapy is used almost exclusively for pain relief, although it may occasionally be used for other conditions. Sometimes when physical therapists such as chiropractors or physiotherapists use this kind of acupuncture in their practice, it is called 'dry needling'.

Traditional Acupuncture, in contrast, is the ancient therapy developed in China, and now widely practised across South East Asia and the world, and is what I am referring to in this book. It is an holistic treatment, based on a fundamentally different way of viewing health and disease. Training courses take around three years. It is probably 'traditional' acupuncture that you think of when you think of acupuncture. It can be used for a very wide range of physical, mental and emotional conditions.

It is my experience (as a traditional acupuncturist) that most people don't realize the huge fundamental difference between these two. Unfortunately, I often meet people who have had medical acupuncture, and found that it hurt a lot, and didn't work, and have then dismissed acupuncture completely. The experience of medical acupuncture being quite painful seems common – this doesn't surprise me, given the amount of training and needling practice that traditional acupuncturists have to go through before they are allowed to practice.

Types of Traditional Acupuncture

The most common style of traditional acupuncture practised all over the world is TCM ('Traditional Chinese Medicine'.) This is what is taught and practised in China, and is the standard for most Western courses in traditional acupuncture. (See page 16 for a discussion of how TCM was created)

Other countries have also developed slightly different styles of their own, for instance Japanese acupuncture is known for its very gentle techniques, and use of hara diagnosis (feeling the abdomen as a diagnostic tool). Korean acupuncture also has slightly different theories, and it tends to favour treating constitutional problems. Some Korean acupuncturists only use acupuncture points on the hands for their treatments. On the whole though, Japanese and Korean acupuncture are quite similar to TCM, although they place less emphasis on the 'deqi' sensation described above.

Auricular acupuncture uses acupuncture points on the ears to treat illness. It can be used alongside other styles (in which case body points will also be used) or on its own. A recent creation – the NADA protocol – uses five acupuncture points on the ear in the treatment of addiction. It is quite easy to teach and practise this simple five-needle protocol, and so it is often practised by nurses or other healthcare providers working with addiction.

Electro-Acupuncture is the name for electrical stimulation to acupuncture needles. The acupuncturist first inserts the needles in the normal way, and then attaches 1 or more pairs of needles to the electro-acupuncture machine via thin cables with clips on the ends. The machine emits regular electric pulses, the frequency and intensity of which can be adjusted by the acupuncturist.

The sensation of electro-acupuncture is not unlike that from a TENS machine. It is quite a strong treatment, and is most often used in the treatment of pain.

5-elements acupuncture was created in the 1950s by an Englishman, JR Worsley. It is sometimes given his name, and called 'Worsley Acupuncture'. It focuses on treating constitutional imbalances, and is said to specialise in psychological and emotional conditions (though these can also be treated by other styles of traditional acupuncture). It is quite different in theory and practice to TCM. It is interesting to note that this particular Worsley style of practice only exists in acupuncture. For instance, there isn't a '5 elements' school of tui na, herbalism, or any other branch of Chinese medicine.

Finally facial rejuvenation acupuncture, or cosmetic acupuncture, is an acupuncture method for reducing the signs of ageing. It can help to reduce wrinkles, tone facial muscles, and improve complexion, as well as working on internal imbalances, just as 'normal' acupuncture does. It provides a natural and side-effect free alternative to botox, chemical peels, fillers and surgical procedures.

Receiving Acupuncture

Once the diagnosis stage is complete, the acupuncturist will draw up a treatment plan, involving a selection of different acupoints, which could be located anywhere on the body. You will normally be asked to lie down on a treatment couch, but it is possible to receive acupuncture in pretty much any relaxed position. Depending on the location of the points to be used, you may be asked to sit, or adopt a different position.

You will normally only have to expose the parts of your body that will be needled. It's best to wear shorts or loose trousers that can be pulled up to access the lower legs, and similarly a loose fitting top, or vest, to expose the arms if necessary.

If you are required to undress further, your acupuncturist should always respect your modesty and privacy. If you feel uncomfortable with anything, you should always say so.

Once you are comfy, the needles will be tapped in and then normally manipulated to achieve 'deqi'. The sensation you feel at each point may be different to the point before, and it may also change over time as you have more treatments.

The needles will be left in for a certain length of time, depending on the desired outcome, and the style of acupuncture being practised. Sometimes they are removed immediately, sometimes left in. For most TCM acupuncture treatments, needles are retained for something like 15-30 minutes. During that time the acupuncturist may go round and re-stimulate the needles once or twice, or they may be left alone.

The main question that I get asked as an acupuncturist is 'does it hurt?' - And the simple answer is 'no'! The initial sensation of needle insertion can sting slightly on sensitive parts of the body, but on less sensitive areas, you may not feel it at all.

The 'deqi' sensation that occurs with the subsequent needle stimulation can be very varied. It is sometimes a little uncomfortable, but almost always better than you would expect!

When the needles are removed, you are unlikely to feel them at all. There is usually no sign afterwards to even show where they have been. Sometimes there will be a little speck of blood, and sometimes a small bruise, but usually neither.

It is possible to feel a little light-headed afterwards, but this soon passes.

Tui Na (Chinese Massage)

Tui na (pronounced 'twee nar', and sometimes known as 'anmo') is an ancient form of Chinese massage therapy which uses the same underlying theory as acupuncture, and can treat a wide range of internal and external conditions. At the moment it is very little known in the UK, and as a tui na practitioner I find myself regularly describing what it is and how it works, as well as how to pronounce it!

It is strange that tui na is not better known, as in China it ranks equally alongside the other branches of Chinese Medicine. It is at least 2000 years old, and many modern massage styles such as Swedish massage and shiatsu are derived from it - shiatsu is essentially tui na's Japanese cousin.

Tui na massage therapists work with both the physical body and the energetic body; They use what you would recognise as massage techniques to ease the knots and tension out of muscles, and at the same time work with the channels and acupoints to regulate and balance the flow of energy (Qi). Sometimes, tui na is called 'acupressure massage' as it uses acupressure, and other manual techniques, to stimulate the same points that are used in acupuncture – but be aware that the term 'acupressure massage' is also applied to other styles of massage, which may or may not be real Chinese tui na!

Tui Na Techniques

There are many different techniques available to the tui na practitioner, and a treatment will normally consist of a selection of different techniques, depending on the circumstances.

Some of these techniques would be instantly recognisable to any massage practitioner such as Rou Fa which is circular kneading, and Ji Fa which is hacking or chopping, however there are a few techniques unique to this therapy. Tui na's 'hallmark' technique is Gun Fa or 'rolling technique' in which the therapist rolls the hand from the knife edge onto the back of the hand and back again in a rhythmic motion. If you find this hard to picture, rest assured it is even harder to perform correctly!

Traditionally, Chinese tui na students were required to practice this important technique on a bag of rice every day for a year before being let loose on a person. These days we are not quite so strict, but rice-bag practice still forms an important part of training.

Another unusual technique which also takes a huge amount of practice to master is Yi Zhi Chan Tui Fa – the beautifully named 'one finger meditation'. The is the tui na therapist's equivalent of the acupuncturist's needle. The thumb is pressed onto an acupoint and then a particular high speed rocking motion is used, in order to stimulate the effects of the point. The therapist focuses their Qi onto the point in a kind of meditation for which the technique is named, thereby bringing about the particular effects of that point.

Styles of Tui Na

Tui na can be broadly divided into Yin and Yang styles. Yin style tui na, sometimes called 'qi gong tui na' is a very gentle healing practice using light touch. It regulates and balances the energy (Qi), clearing stagnation and strengthening organ function. It is a deeply calming and relaxing treatment and is suitable for all internal conditions, stress management and for those who prefer a light touch or who dislike strong massage. Practitioners of this style of tui na need to be able to effectively work with Qi, and to this end are normally chi kung or t'ai chi practitioners as well.

Yang style tui na is a more physical treatment that uses deep penetrating techniques to break down muscular tension. It is extremely effective on knots and tight muscles, but without being painful as some deep massages can be. It is similar to deep tissue massage or sports massage, and is very effective for pain relief and very tense or knotted muscles.

Sometimes tui na is described as a very strong, vigorous massage by those who are not familiar with the Yin style of practice. In actual fact, a skilled and well trained practitioner will use both Yin and Yang techniques as required, and most treatments are somewhere between the 2 extremes. There are no set routines, and treatments are always tailored to each person depending on individual needs.

What Can Tui Na Treat?

The theory of tui na is the same as that of acupuncture, so it has the same detailed diagnostic methods and complex understanding of the body and mind. This is what marks it as separate from most other massage. In tui na, the therapy is inseparable from the theory.

This makes tui na suitable for far more than just muscular problems, and it can be successfully used for a range of health problems and conditions including respiratory, circulatory, digestive, psycho-emotional and hormonal problems to name a few. In fact, it can be considered a kind of 'acupuncture without needles'. It is also of great benefit in maintaining health and dealing with stress.

Receiving Tui Na

Tui na is traditionally performed through material, so you will normally not be required to undress, although you may be asked to remove some clothing if you are wearing lots of layers, or anything particularly bulky or which would get in the way of the treatment. Depending on what you're wearing, you may also prefer to remove some clothing for reasons of comfort. Normally tui na practitioners will cover you over with a thin piece of soft material called a tui na cloth to make application of the techniques easier.

You may well receive part or all of your tui na treatment lying on a treatment couch. Quite possibly your practitioner will ask you to move into different positions at different times to get to different part of your body. You may also receive treatment sat in a chair. There are many different ways of working, and if any particular positions are difficult or uncomfortable for you, then you should say so, and your practitioner will be able to work around that.

The treatment may include certain manipulations or stretches. If your tui na practitioner moves, twists or stretches any part of your body, you should relax as much as possible. Resist the urge to 'help' and instead, unless directed otherwise, go limp and floppy like a rag doll to allow the full application of the technique.

Yang style tui na, which uses stronger, more penetrating techniques, can be uncomfortable and tender, but should never be outright painful. You should always tell your practitioner if anything hurts.

Chapter 10

Nutrition And Herbalism – The Energetic Properties Of Plants

ENERGETICS VS CHEMICAL CONSTITUENTS

It's pretty obvious that a chilli pepper is a 'hot' food, but would you have thought that lamb and trout are too? Or that seaweed and mango are very Cold?

According to the principles of Chinese medicine all foods and herbs can be categorized according to their energetic temperature, whether they are Cold, Cool, Neutral, Warm or Hot. What this describes is the effect of the food on the body, quite simply, what it does to you when you eat it. This is in keeping with the holistic view of Chinese Medicine, but somewhat at odds with standard Western ideas.

For instance, the fact that a banana is high in potassium, with abundant fibre and vitamins C and B6 is largely irrelevant to a traditional Chinese medical practitioner, as these concepts do not form a part of the medical framework in which he or she is working. However, the knowledge that bananas are Cold & Sweet and nourish Yin has immediate relevance – for a person who has a diagnosis of Yin Deficiency, is on the Warm and Dry side, and who maybe suffers from constipation, bananas would be an ideal food. On the other hand, for the Cold, Damp individual bananas might aggravate an existing condition.

This is not to say that knowing the chemical make-up of a food or herb has no value, and indeed the modern practitioner will often make use of this information, but using the traditional energetic descriptions of foods and herbs aligns the understanding of them with the Chinese diagnosis and treatment plan.

Foods and herbs are described not only by their temperature but also by their flavours, routes and actions.

The 5 flavours relate to the 5 elements of Chinese Medicine, and also to different organs:

- Salty relates to Water and the Kidneys, it regulates fluid in the body and encourages movement inwards and downwards. It softens and detoxifies.

- Sour relates to Wood and the Liver and has an astringent effect, encouraging contraction and absorption. The sour flavour helps to overcome stagnation.

- Bitter relates to Fire and the Heart, and has a draining and drying effect. It is of most use in excessive Patterns and is reduced for those who are Cold and/or Deficient.

- Sweet relates to Earth and the Spleen. It is the most building and nourishing flavour. Note that this refers to the natural sweet flavour as found in root vegetables and grains (Refined sweeteners such as sugar, although clearly very sweet, do not have the same nourishing effect)

- Pungent relates to Metal and the Lung. It promotes the circulation of Qi and Blood, dispersing stagnation.

Finally, the 'route' of a food or herb is which channel (meridian) is effected, and the 'action' describes any other therapeutic effect, for instance if it tonifies Qi, clears pathogenic Heat, or aids Blood circulation. The combination of temperature, flavour route and actions gives us a complete overview of exactly how that substance will affect the body and mind when taken.

Dietary Therapy / Nutrition

When Hippocrates said "Let thy food be thy medicine and thy medicine be thy food" a few hundred years BC he wouldn't have known it but he was saying the same thing as Chinese doctors of the time – who proposed that food and medicine share the same source.

And the beauty of the using food as medicine, is that we all need to eat. As you have seen, your Qi and Blood is manufactured out of the Qi of the food that you eat, so what and how you eat has an enormous effect on your whole system.

The digestive process, under the control of the Spleen and Stomach, is called the 'centre' – it is at the centre of our physical body, and also it is at the centre of the Qi production mechanism. Regardless of what your imbalance is, or what condition you are suffering from, an ample supply of Qi and Blood, and a strong unhindered digestive system is essential. Hence the advice in Chinese medicine that above all else you must always 'protect the centre'.

In ancient China dietary therapy was considered the first treatment of choice for most conditions and only if this failed to have any results were other methods such as acupuncture, herbs or tui na massage administered.

In modern China today the regular use of medicinal foods survives among the population in a far more sophisticated way than our 'an apple a day keeps the doctor away'! In fact, medicinal ingredients are regularly cooked into soups and other dishes to maintain health and well-being – a practice that I am also doing my best to spread around my patients, clients and students!

General Guidelines

Chinese medicine recommends a 'light, clear' diet, consisting of whole grains and vegetables, lightly cooked (e.g. steamed or stir-fried) with a little meat, fruit and nuts and seeds. Heavy, rich and processed foods should be kept to a bare minimum as they introduce pathogenic Heat and Dampness into the system.

The preparation and cooking of food is also important to its energetic qualities. One of the distinct contrasts to commonly held Western ideas is to do with the relative merits of cold, raw food. In Chinese thought, cold and raw foods such as salads, smoothies and raw fruit are considered Cold in energetic nature and quite detoxifying. They are thus suitable for strong, robust, Hot natured people but not really recommended in large amounts for frail, Cold or weak people, or those with digestive difficulties.

Because it takes so much more energy to digest cold and raw food, anyone with digestive problems such as food intolerance, bloating, IBS, indigestion etc. would be wise to move to more cooked and warm foods. Slow cooked soups, stews and casseroles are all excellent choices for most of us, as they are the easiest foods to digest, and reach the stomach in a state where their Qi can easily be utilised.

This doesn't mean that all cold and raw food is bad, as some acupuncturists may tell you, but simply that it is not appropriate for everyone in large amounts. In fact, there is really no such thing as a bad food, it's a case of understanding the energetics of a food, and then deciding whether or not it is appropriate for you at the current time.

The way you eat is also important – you should eat in a calm and relaxed environment, enjoying and focusing on your food. If you are distracted, for instance if you eat in front of television or whilst reading, then your digestion suffers. Sadly, fewer and fewer of us really take pleasure in food and modern life dictates that we must eat 'on the run'. However, if you can, eating sitting at a table and taking time to enjoy your food allows your Qi to do its work un-distracted and your digestion will benefit.

In line with a slower pace of eating is the recommendation to chew your food '100 times' or 'until it is water'. Of course, it is the chewing of food and mixing it with saliva that is the first stage in the digestive process. Next time you have something to eat count how many times you chew. While 100 chews may be a little extreme the idea of chewing your food more is worth consideration.

The advice 'eat breakfast like a king, lunch like a prince, and dinner like a pauper' exists in many cultures, and also forms an important part of the Chinese view. The digestive system is at its strongest from 7-11am and at its weakest from 7-11pm, so it is wise to have a large breakfast and a small evening meal (ideally no later than 7pm). For those looking to lose weight this is doubly important – if any further proof were needed bear in mind that Japanese sumo wrestlers do the opposite and eat massive meals late in the evening in order to maintain their weight!

Specific Advice

Beyond these basic guidelines, a practitioner of Chinese Nutritional (or 'Dietary') Therapy will be able to recommend specific foods and cooking methods, as well as giving you further advice on exactly what and how to eat, depending on your exact diagnosis.

As with all the other branches of Chinese medicine, exactly what kinds of foods are good to eat, and which are not, depends on your own personal state of health at the time. This is a very important point, which is often overlooked when it comes to food. As I have said, there is no such thing as a 'good' food. All there is, is suitable or unsuitable at this current time. What's good for you might not be good for me.

This is obvious, when you think about it, but the idea of foods that are good for you, and foods that aren't, is so common that it's hard to avoid. This way of thinking puts all the 'goodness' or 'badness' in the food, but ignores the fact that every person is unique and has different requirements. In fact, whether a food is suitable or not is to do with the interaction between the nature of the food, the season and environment, and your own constitution and current state of health.

Nutrition In Practice

There are many ways of working with diet and nutrition, and all nutritional therapists work slightly differently.

You may well be asked to keep a food diary as a way of assessing your current diet. This can be a very useful process, as it highlights exactly what you're eating. Often just the act of keeping a food diary makes you realise that your diet is not as balanced or healthy as you thought it was!

Your practitioner may also recommend one or more food 'experiments' – for instance, cutting out a certain food or kind of food for a certain period. This is a good way to check for intolerances.

Some Western trained nutritional therapists use a lot of supplements, but I do not believe that this is a particularly useful way of working. Supplements have their place, but high dose supplements or combinations of lots of different supplements can cause problems of their own, and can be dangerous. In my opinion, it is much better to work naturally, with food.

Herbalism

Chinese herbalism has become well known all around the world, but there is often some confusion about what kinds of substances herbalists use, and the manner in which they are used.

For a start the common term 'herbalism' is very misleading, as Chinese herbalists would traditionally use a range of different healing substances, not just 'herbs'. The vast majority of these would be parts of plants, including roots, stems, flowers, fruits, seeds and bark. As well as plants, certain minerals, shells and other substances are used.

Some of these 'herbs' are things you might recognise, such as dried ginger, chrysanthemum flower, or mint, but most you're unlikely to know. Most controversial is the use of animal parts. Traditionally, certain animal parts such as tiger bones were used medicinally, but these days absolutely no parts from endangered species are used by reputable practitioners, either in China or outside.

Some parts from *non*-endangered animals may still be used in some countries, and some are parts that do not require the animal to be killed such as deer-antler velvet or shed snake skin. However, such is the strong feeling against using animal parts in the UK, and other parts of Europe that even these sustainable animal parts are not used in modern practice by many Chinese herbalists. If in doubt, check with the practitioner before you go to see them, and they should be happy to explain their position to you.

Chinese Herbal prescriptions are complex, and may often involve a dozen or more ingredients. Chinese herbalists rarely use herbs individually, as the interaction between the different herbs in a formula is very important, with some herbs added to support the effect of the other ingredients, to harmonise the blend, or to make it more digestible, for example.

Many ancient formulas dating back thousands of years are still in use today, and may form the basis of a prescription, which is then modified depending on individual requirements and diagnosis.

The herbs would traditionally have been used loose, and boiled up in batches to make a kind of 'tea', enough for one or two days. If you are given boil-up herbs you will probably be given a number of bags, to make enough for a week or two. Once you've had these, you will check in with your practitioner, who will either give you more bags the same, or modify the prescription if necessary.

Instead of the traditional 'boil-up' herbs, you may be given a tub of concentrated herbal powder to dissolve in water to make a tea, or capsules or tablets which are easier, and not as unpleasant tasting, but are sometimes considered less effective than the raw 'boil-up' herbs.

While a qualified herbalist is able to make up formulas for each individual, there are also many well known standard formulas which are available ready-made in tablet form – these are often known as 'patent medicines'. They are available over the counter, and the Chinese regularly self-prescribe using patent medicines in much the same way as we might go to the chemist and get a box of aspirin or some cough syrup without a professional prescription. They are also used by qualified practitioners for their convenience and time-tested effectiveness.

Unfortunately the current situation in the UK prohibits the sale of herbal patent medicines, following an EU directive that came into force in 2011. This is an enormous shame, and severely limits the use of Chinese herbal medicines in this country. The situation is not fixed, and may change in the future, but for the time being patent medicines are not available anywhere in the UK.

Western Herbs

In fact, there is no reason why a Chinese Herbalist must limit him or herself to the use of Chinese herbs. Some practitioners, myself included, are drawn to making use of the plants that grow around us, rather than those on the other side of the globe. This doesn't mean abandoning Chinese medical principles, as we can use Western herbs in a Chinese way – in other words, by using them according to their energetic properties, and within the framework of Chinese Medicine.

This is a way of saying that it is the way that herbs are used that makes the difference between Western or Chinese herbal medicine, not where the herbs happen to grow. In fact, Chinese medicine makes use of herbs that are not native to China, just as Western herbalists use herbs from China and all over the world.

Just like with food, it is the energetics that are important in Chinese medicine, not the chemical constituents. So Western herbs like parsley and rosemary can be classified by their energetic temperature, flavour, route and action, just as Chinese herbs can, and when used this way, fit perfectly into a Chinese medical treatment.

Chapter 11

T'ai Chi and Chi Kung

Exercising the Qi

While most westerners have heard of t'ai chi (or 'tai-ji'), the term chi kung (or 'qi gong') is still less well known. In practice, the 2 are very closely related, and the boundaries are blurred. Chi kung means something like 'energy work' and is actually quite a broad term which includes t'ai chi, so technically t'ai chi is a kind of chi kung.

In any case, t'ai chi and chi kung are ancient practices normally involving specific movements, breathing techniques and mental devices such as visualisation or meditation. There are many different styles, and practices vary hugely between one and another.

You might recognise t'ai chi as the slow graceful movements practised by elderly Chinese in parks or other public areas in the mornings – this is a common occurrence anywhere that there are a few Chinese families living nearby.

The exercises of chi kung or t'ai chi normally consist of a number of slow movements in sequence combined with specific breathing techniques, and sometimes visualisations. Sometimes no movements are used, especially in meditation exercises. Most styles have many different exercises for different purposes.

One of the distinguishing factors between t'ai chi and chi kung is that t'ai chi generally has one or more long sets of movements or 'forms', and chi kung tends to consist or smaller or simpler movements. The t'ai chi forms may consist of many hundreds of movements, each one flowing into the next. The longest forms can take years to learn, and a lifetime to master! During practice the aim is to concentrate completely on the movements, and empty the mind of distractions. For this reason it is often called 'meditation in motion'.

Styles of Chi Kung and T'ai Chi

First references to these ancient arts appear in ancient Chinese texts. The Chinese philosopher Zhuang Zi, writing in 600 BCE said 'breathing techniques can improve metabolism; moving like a bear and a bird will result in longevity'. Around 250 BCE the famous Taoist doctor Hua To created the '5 animal play' chi kung in which mimicking animal movements was said to balance the 5 elements and improve health and well-being.

Since then chi kung and t'ai chi has multiplied, developed, and spread across the globe. There is now a bewildering range of styles available, covering all aspects of health, martial arts, and self-cultivation.

Chi kung is typically divided into 5 types: Taoist, Buddhist, Confucian, Medical & Martial, however, these are broad distinctions and many styles fall into more than 1 category. In fact, Confucian chi kung is rare, and most types of chi kung and t'ai chi can be traced back to either Buddhist or Taoist roots.

Pretty much all chi kung and t'ai chi has overall health maintenance as one of its main aims. The exercises involved both regulate and strengthen the Qi, and benefit overall health and well-being, as well as being deeply relaxing. Medical chi kung specifically focuses on this aspect and deals with the treatment of illness.

Martial types of chi kung and t'ai chi are the least focussed on healing, as you may expect, and instead they concentrate on developing fighting and self defence skills. Some t'ai chi styles practice a partner exercise called 'push hands' which develops sensitivity to your own body movements, and those of your partner, and these skills can easily be applied in martial situations. Similarly, some styles of chi kung like the famous 'iron shirt' style practise tough body conditioning techniques in order that practitioners can better withstand blows and strikes. These are often called 'hard' or 'external' styles, as opposed to the 'soft' or 'internal' styles which are less concerned with the physical body, and more with the internal aspect of Qi.

Chi kung and t'ai chi form the backbone of the Chinese yang sheng or self-cultivation techniques. Most chi kung practitioners notice better health, improved posture, deeper breathing and a calmer more positive outlook. With dedicated practice, spiritual development can be pursued, if desired; Most chi kung and t'ai chi, and certainly the Taoist types, is seen as a form of self development in which the physical, mental, emotional and spiritual spheres are all improved through practice.

Clinical Uses of T'ai Chi and Chi Kung

The use of chi kung skills in a clinical or therapeutic setting by a Chinese medicine practitioner is sometimes called 'medical chi kung' and it overlaps greatly with Yin style tui na.

In chi kung treatment, a master chi kung practitioner can use their own Qi to influence yours. There are many ways to do this – you may be asked to lie, sit or stand in a certain position, and the practitioner may make gentle contact with you, or may remain 'hands-off'.

Skilled Yin style tui na specialists work in much the same way, first of all getting into the 'chi kung state' and connecting with their own Qi, before making a connection with you.

They may also touch or press certain acupoints, or hold different parts of your body. You may be asked to breathe in a certain way, or perform some kind of visualisation.

During this kind of treatment you will normally feel very relaxed. You may be aware of a 'Qi sensation' in your body, for instance a warmth, tingling or sensation of movement. Occasionally you might feel a stronger sensation, or have an emotional reaction as old blockages are cleared.

This can be a deep and profound healing practice, and it relies almost entirely on the degree of chi kung mastery of the practitioner. It is an advanced way of working, and takes a great deal of dedicated self-cultivation on behalf of the practitioner - as chi kung is a self-cultivation practice, you should look for a practitioner who appears to have achieved a certain degree of advancement in this area - This is not easy to judge, but I would suggest as a minimum they should be relaxed, humble, easy-going, and generally healthy.

Even if you do not practice t'ai chi or chi kung, or receive a chi kung treatment, a good Chinese medicine practitioner will be able to teach you aspects of these arts to do at home – for instance a deep breathing exercise, meditation or relaxation technique. This can be a very important part of your overall treatment 'package'.

Chapter 12

Supplementary Treatments

In addition to the 5 main branches of Chinese medicine, there are a host of supplementary treatments and techniques which practitioners can call upon. These 'supplementary' treatments can be used on their own, but are normally combined with other forms of treatment, particularly acupuncture. The most common of these are moxa (or 'moxibustion'), cupping and gua sha.

Moxa

Moxibustion is the name given to the burning of Chinese

Mugwort (or Moxa) in order to provide a gentle source of heat to an acupoint or body part. It is often used for conditions involving Cold and/or Stagnation.

Moxa is very versatile, and can be used in a number of ways, and it can be focused on one specific point or used on a large area. The sensation can be of a very mild warmth, through to quite a strong heat. It is normally quite pleasant to receive.

Traditional moxa produces a great deal of strongly scented smoke when it burns, and some practitioners find this a problem – it certainly causes issues if it's used a great deal. There's absolutely no way you can use moxa in any amount in a room that doesn't have ventilation, for instance.

For this reason, smokeless moxa is quite popular. This is a kind of moxa-infused charcoal, which burns slowly, emits no smoke and has only a faint smell. Smokeless moxa can be used on almost any occasion where traditional moxa can.

Moxa Stick

A moxa stick is a roll of tightly packed moxa wrapped in paper – something like a cigar. Smokeless moxa sticks are also commonly used. The practitioner lights the end of the stick and then brings it close to the body. Sometimes this is used to stimulate an acupoint, and sometimes the stick is moved along the length of a channel or over part of the body. The level of heat is easily adjusted by moving the stick closer to the body or further away, making this a versatile way of working.

Warming Needle

First of all, a metal-handled needle is inserted into an

acupoint by the acupuncturist. Then, a ball of loose moxa, a slice of moxa-stick or a ready-made piece of moxa is placed on the end of the needle's handle and lit. As it burns, the needle heats up and the heat is transferred into the body through the needle. This provides a relatively gentle heat.

Indirect Moxa

The practitioner fashions a cone of loose moxa by squeezing and rolling it between his or her fingers, or uses a ready made cone or small piece of smokeless moxa, and places it on the body, on top of an insulating material (to prevent burns)

The insulating material can be inert, or can add therapeutic value. For instance, a slice of root ginger is traditionally used, as it adds a further warming effect to the treatment. Flat dried 'cakes' of powdered herbs and water can also be used. Normally a number of cones of moxa are used one after another.

This is a very traditional way of using moxa, but now less common than the other methods, possibly because more preparation is required. The heat from indirect moxa builds up gradually, and can get quite strong.

Direct Moxa

Direct moxa is probably the least commonly used in modern practice. In this style, a moxa cone is placed directly on the skin and lit. It is removed as it begins to burn down close to the skin, and normally a few cones are used one after the other. For direct moxa the cones are normally quite small, and sometimes only tiny rice-grain sized 'threads' of moxa are used, which makes it easier to control the level of heat. Direct moxa has a strong effect, with a strong penetrating heat.

Scarring Moxa

By far the strongest treatment possible with moxa, so called 'scarring' moxa is direct moxa where the cone is allowed to burn down to the skin. This method deliberately burns the skin, and creates a scar. As the scar heals, it is like a constant stimulation of the acupoint, providing a strong therapeutic effect.

Needless to say, this method of using moxa has all but disappeared, at least in the West, although it used to be very common in China.

There is a real technique to carrying out scarring moxa, and few practitioners are trained in its administration. Rest assured, that there is no occasion where scarring moxa is essential, and it is included in this book more for the sake of interest and completeness than because you'll be encountering it as part of your treatment!

Cupping

Another common accompaniment to acupuncture or tui na is cupping. This technique involves the use of glass or plastic 'cups' which are placed onto the body after a partial vacuum is first created inside using a flame or a suction gun. This causes the cup to stick to the body.

The technique for using cups is quite simple, and it is often used as a folk medicine not only in China but also across Europe. Families in China often use empty jam jars for cupping each other!

The effects of this technique are to stimulate circulation of the area and relax tense muscles. It can also be used to 'draw out pathogens' in the case of Wind Invasion (common cold, flu etc.) especially when used on the back.

There are a few ways to use cups. Stationary cupping involves placing the cups and leaving them in place for a while. Slide cupping involves putting the cups on the body with a little oil and sliding them from one place to another to cover a larger area. Finally, flash cupping is where the cups are placed on the body and then quickly removed, in order to provide a milder stimulation.

Cupping is not at all painful, but be aware that it does leave bruises. Strong cupping can leave dark bruises that take a few days or a week to fade. This makes it look like quite a drastic treatment, when in fact, it is relatively mild!

Gua Sha

Gua sha or 'scraping' is less commonly practiced by Western therapists, but has always been an important therapeutic technique for Chinese medicine practitioners. It is mainly used by tui na practitioners and acupuncturists. Gua sha is used where there is stagnation, and can often be helpful for pain.

First of all a little oil is applied to the area to be treated, and then a special tool (little more than a flat piece of plastic or stone) is used to gently scrape the skin until a Sha forms. The Sha is a red, rash-like appearance on the skin which indicates that the gua sha treatment has been effective.

Like cupping, gua sha looks like a strong treatment, and the rash-like sha can appear to be quite severe, when in fact gua sha is not unpleasant to receive. Like a bruise, the sha normally fades within a few days.

Other Supplementary Therapies

As well as moxa, cupping and gua sha, there are innumerable additional therapies that practitioner can draw on.

You may encounter the topical use of herbs – either as a lotion or herbal oil, or a compress or patch of herbs applied to the skin. Tui na practitioners are particularly likely to use oils and lotions, even if the bulk of the tui na treatment is carried out the traditional way, through clothes. For instance, they may apply a little herbal oil or lotion at the end of the treatment.

Electric heat lamps are a simple way of warming an area, and are often used as an easy alternative to moxa. They are used extensively in Chinese hospitals (where they are sometimes called 'magic lamps'!) and practitioners who have trained in China will often use them.

Chapter 13

After Your Treatment

All the branches of Chinese medicine are holistic, and work on your overall health on physical, mental and emotional levels. As you strengthen and regulate your Qi, eliminate blockages and restore balance, you will notice improvements in your overall well-being in many ways.

I call these improvements 'positive side-effects'. They can include more energy, better sleep, or a feeling of calmness. No matter what you are having treatment for, you should notice improvements like these as your system becomes stronger and more efficient.

If you are having acupuncture or tui na treatment, you may notice some soreness or tenderness following treatment in the areas that have been worked on, this is especially true with strong Yang style tui na. This kind of soreness can be worse the following day, but should not last more than a day or two. With more gentle tui na, and quite often with acupuncture, there is no soreness or tenderness at all.

If you have made dietary adjustments, or are taking new herbs or foods, they should be well tolerated. If you experience any digestive upsets, or anything that could indicate an allergic reaction, notify your practitioner immediately.

One of the aims of any kind of Chinese medicine is to clear blockages. Sometimes, the effects of this clearing manifest on an emotional or mental level. When this happens it is as if the emotion has been 'released' and you can feel especially happy, sad, angry, or whatever the emotion is that has been blocked or trapped. This 'releasing' of trapped emotions is very beneficial, and you should do your best to simply allow it to happen without judgement or analysis – the emotion will come and go in its own time.

Similarly on a mental level, you may notice that following treatment you notice a mental shift – maybe an experience of the 'penny dropping', or that you are able to make connections where you could not before, or that your concentration is clearer.

On the whole, you should feel good following your treatment! Negative or unpleasant effects are rare, but if you do notice anything, you should inform your practitioner.

Section 4

Maintenance, Prevention and 'Nourishing Life'

Chapter 14

Step 3 of 3 - Cultivate Radiant Health

Once your diagnosis and the main body of your treatment are complete, and your condition is treated, or under control, you move on to Step 3 of the '3 Steps To Radiant Health', which I call 'Cultivate Radiant Health'.

There are really 3 parts to this step of treatment:

1. Maintain Health Gains

Depending on your individual circumstances, you may need maintenance or 'top-up' treatments in order to maintain the improvements you have seen. This is particularly the case when there is a structural element to the condition, for instance, the bony growths of osteoarthritis, or unrepairable damage resulting from a serious accident.

In these kinds of cases, maintenance treatment is normally best at roughly monthly intervals, occasionally slightly longer.

2. Prevent Future Illness

There are enormous benefits to going for regular treatments when you are well, and/or your condition is under control. It is tempting to think that the work is done – you were unwell, and now you are well – but this is to stop short and miss out on so much more. For one thing, regular treatment makes it possible to spot any potential problems well in advance and nip them in the bud.

Your practitioner will be able to use the Chinese diagnostic tools described in Section 2 to spot the signs of an imbalance before it becomes too pronounced or 'takes hold'. In this way, the chances of suffering from both minor and more serious health conditions is minimised.

Again, treatments for prevention purposes are best about monthly.

3. Continually Improve Health And Well-Being

Maintenance and prevention are great, but there is always a place for a helping hand in the continual journey towards 'Radiant Health'.

Radiant Health is a state of full and joyous engagement with life on all levels. It includes physical health and fitness, a strong and flexible body, good immunity, a clear mind and sharp concentration. It is also about a feeling of contentment, emotional balance, adaptability and peace.

This is a powerful concept that goes far beyond simply removing or treating an illness or condition. It is a life-long journey of self-cultivation, moving towards an optimum state of physical, mental, emotional and spiritual well-being. 'Health' can be defined as the absence of disease, but of course you can be free from disease but still not feel good. Radiant Health, on the other hand, is a state where you are free from disease, and feel great!

For me, this is the goal of the whole of Chinese Medicine – the continuation of the journey towards Radiant Health. I call it a journey, because it is all about the constant and gradual movement in the right direction – away from illness and towards Radiant Health. You may at this moment be quite well, or you may be quite unwell. It doesn't matter. Where-ever you are, you can use the tools and techniques of Chinese Medicine to move away from illness and towards Radiant Health.

These days we tend to think of Chinese medicine as something to use when we get sick or ill – in just the same way as we use modern Western medicine. But this is to miss one of the greatest strengths of the Chinese system. In fact, all the different branches and practices contained within Chinese medicine can and should be used for health maintenance, prevention of illness, personal development and self-cultivation.

You don't need to have a specific 'illness' or 'condition' to benefit from this kind of treatment, and even if you first go for help with a particular problem, you don't have to stop once you are 'better', because, chances are, there are still plenty of areas where you could be 'better still'!

Chapter 15

Yang Sheng - Nourishing Life

My first introduction to Chinese medicine was not in the form of a treatment, but through t'ai chi practice, and as I learnt about the Chinese theories of health, my first thought was how I could apply them to myself. Although I didn't know the term at the time, I was learning and practising 'yang sheng'.

The term 'yang sheng' means 'nourishing life', a concept that has always played an important part in Chinese Medicine. Yang sheng includes specific health-promoting and self-cultivation practices, and philosophies and guidelines for a long and healthy life, mainly derived from Taoist thought.

As well as treatments you can receive, the 5 branches of Chinese medicine are all things you can also do for yourself, with the obvious exception of acupuncture, unless you are trained in it! Some training and guidance in this area may well form part of your treatment plan, especially in step 3, the maintenance and development phase of your treatment.

I have personally experienced the benefits of this approach, and so I've introduced this important element of Chinese Medicine into my practice – I do as much teaching, coaching and training as I do treatment.

Skilled Chinese medicine practitioners have worked this way throughout history, teaching their patients specific exercises they can do at home, demonstrating breathing techniques, explaining stress reduction methods, and discussing diet. This is a powerful way of working. Not only does it provide a way for you to 'top up' in-between visits, it is also very empowering. Learning these kinds of techniques is a way of taking control of your health and well-being.

Here is a list of just some of the tools available in the 'Yang Sheng Toolbox' which you can do yourself at home

Chi Kung (Qi Gong)

This ranges from full t'ai chi forms that take years to learn, down to simple breathing exercises or channel (meridian) stretches. It also incorporates various de-stressing techniques and meditations. If you don't want to take up a full t'ai chi or chi kung practice, or don't have time, then it is still possible to benefit from this powerful branch of yang sheng and Chinese medicine, just by learning and practising some simple techniques.

For instance, most adults unwittingly adopt poor breathing habits, and use only a small portion of their lung capacity. Breathing becomes shallow and rapid, instead of slow and deep. It also rises up to the top section of the lungs instead of sinking down towards the belly. Learning how to use deep abdominal breathing is itself an amazingly effective health and well-being practice, and something I regularly teach to my clients and students.

Acupressure & Self-Massage

The art of self-massage and acupressure is occasionally called 'anmo gong'. It can be used on its own as a daily health and well-being practice, incorporated into a wider treatment plan for a specific condition, or used as an occasional 'remedy' for minor complaints.

There are many tui na massage techniques that can effectively be used on yourself, and most of the acupoints are accessible for acupressure or other manual stimulation techniques, for instance rubbing or tapping – there are really only a few on the back which you can't get to. This makes it quite possible to give yourself virtually a full acupressure/tui na treatment.

Over the years I have developed a number of acupressure / self-tui na routines for different purposes. They are enjoyable and simple to do, and have a great benefit, and I make them part of my regular practice.

Nutrition / Diet

Needless to say, this is something that is rarely done for or to you, but something you do for yourself. For the most part, you decide what, how and when you eat, which is exactly what makes diet such a very useful and effective form of medicine.

Your Qi and Blood are manufactured primarily from the building blocks provided by the food you eat, and eating a good diet, and one that is suited to your individual circumstances, is one of the best ways of improving health.

Herbs

Just like all of the branches of Chinese medicine, herbs can be used not only to treat illness but also for 'Yang-Sheng' self-cultivation purposes. The tonic herbs are particularly effective in this area. There are a range of Chinese and Western herbs that can be used either in cooking or in supplement form to strengthen and regulate the whole system, or address specific imbalances.

In China herbs are regularly used in cooking to impart therapeutic or tonic properties to the dish. This is a practice I would like to encourage us to take up here in the UK!

Lifestyle Considerations

Yang sheng principles are derived from Taoist thought, and a large part of yang sheng is to do with 'going with the flow' and following the way of nature.

In part, this means following the rhythms and cycles of nature – which we have become almost completely detached from in the past few generations, now that most of us have little need to be attached to the land or the seasons.

In general terms, this means being more active and 'outward focused' in the Spring and Summer, and quieter, more restful and 'inward focused' in the Autumn and Winter. The same applies for the day and night cycle.

It also means re-connecting with the natural world, and following the Taoist path of yielding and non-resistance. This is a gentle way of life that avoids direct confrontation, and following the natural ebbs and flows. This is a big subject in itself – for more information try one of the books in the resources section.

Non-Chinese Yang Sheng

Finally, anything that nourishes your life and benefits health and well-being can be considered a form of yang sheng. This might be social gatherings with friends and family, walking in the woods, or artistic pursuits.

It also includes yoga, 'internal' martial arts, and religious or spiritual activities among other practices.

For more free information and resources
on yang sheng practice, visit:

www.neilkingham.com

Section 5

Final Thoughts And Resources

Chapter 16

Putting It All Together

In the preceding pages, I have taken you on a whistle-stop tour of the practice of Chinese medicine, from diagnosis, through treatment, and to maintenance and health-cultivation. The aim has been to show you what a Chinese medicine treatment consists of, as well as something of the how and why behind it.

I present here one final case study, to illustrate these principles in practice.

Case Study: Simon

Simon is in his late 30s, and first came to me complaining of stress, difficulty sleeping, and eczema. Simon runs a small business, and works long hours. He describes himself as 'always on the go'. His health had always been good, but in recent years he had found that his energy was less, and he was starting to notice a lot of minor niggles and health problems that had never bothered him before.

On questioning, Simon said that he sometimes had a sensation of fluttering in the chest, and his sleep was restless and dream-disturbed. He tended to be on the hot side, especially at night. He said he had trouble switching off and relaxing, and that his mind was always busy.

His pulse was rapid, thin and weak, and his tongue was deeply cracked, with a red tip.

Step 1 - Diagnosis:

The red patches of eczema, feeling hot, and being 'always on the go' suggested a Pattern of Heat which was confirmed by Simon's rapid pulse. The fact that he was mainly hot at night (the most 'Yin' time of day) and had dream disturbed sleep, plus lots of cracks in his tongue and a thin and weak pulse, refines this diagnosis to Empty Heat (Yin Deficiency.) Finally, the red tip of the tongue and palpitations, along with the other signs and symptoms, told me that the Heart is involved. So, Simon's main diagnosis is Heart Yin Deficiency.

Step 2 - Treatment:

I initially saw Simon weekly, using a combination of acupuncture and yin style tui na to help him to relax. I chose acupoints that had a calming, grounding effect and which would strengthen Yin. He immediately noticed feeling calmer and more relaxed following our sessions.

I also taught him a simple deep-breathing exercise to practice at home, and we discussed some small dietary alterations that would help such as drinking plenty of water, and reducing his coffee intake. Over the next few weeks I also introduced some more specific dietary advice based on reducing heating foods and increasing yin-tonic foods.

After a month, Simon reported that he was feeling much more grounded and in-control in work, and felt more able to deal with stressful situations. His sleep was a little better and energy levels higher. He felt there might have been a little bit of improvement in his eczema, but not much.

At this point, I prescribed a herbal skin cream for the eczema, and as he was enjoying doing the breathing exercise so much and found it so useful, I also taught him a slightly more advanced version of the exercise, and some acupressure techniques he could use himself.

Another month on, and Simon told me he was a 'new man'. He felt far more relaxed and less stressed, was sleeping much better, and had more energy. The eczema was still there, but considerably reduced.

Step 3 – Maintenance

At that point, we decided to switch to fortnightly sessions, which we gradually expanded to 3 weeks apart, and then monthly. I still see Simon once every 4-6 weeks, and am very pleased to say that all the symptoms that he came with are well under control, and he feels he has a new lease of life. Now, when he has a stressful time at work he is able to take it in his stride, and knows the techniques that will stop the stress from effecting his sleep.

We continue to work together to keep this going, to further improve Simon's health and well-being on all levels, and to identify and prevent any future illness before it happens.

Glossary

I have deliberately used as few technical terms and as little Chinese as possible throughout this book for the sake of readability. This short glossary should help to 'fill in the gaps' in case you come across a term that you don't understand, or haven't encountered before.

3 Treasures – The three essential aspects or energies that make up human life – Jing, Qi and Shen.

5 Elements – The 5 elements, or 5 phases, are Water, Wood, Fire, Earth and Metal. They are a way of describing 5 states of being, and they are used to categorise the organs along with their corresponding emotions, sounds, colours, flavours and so on. Also the name of a particular style of acupuncture (see page 109)

6 Divisions – A theoretical and therapeutic framework that pairs the 12 channels, giving 6 'divisions'. The 6 divisions are called Tai Yang, Shao Yang, Yang Ming, Tai Yin, Shao Yin and Jue Yin.

8 Principles – An important diagnostic tool, categorising an illness or condition on the basis of 4 pairs of opposites (see page 43)

Anmo – An old name for tui na.

Constitutional Factor (CF) - A term used by 5-elements style acupuncturists, referring to the idea of one main constitutional imbalance, expressed as one of the five elements. For instance, you may be a 'Fire CF' if your main constitutional imbalance is in the Fire element. The term is not used outside of this specific style of acupuncture.

Chi Kung – A form of Chinese exercise, related to t'ai chi. See Chapter 11.

Ching – An alternate spelling for Jing, rarely used.

Cun - A unit of measurement, based on proportional body size, and used to locate acupoints.

Dampness – Pathological fluid, can cause heaviness, tiredness and oedema. See page 65.

Dao – Alternate spelling of Tao.

Du – The Chinese name for one of the extra vessels, also called the Governing Vessel. See page 106.

Empty Cold – Another name for Yang Deficiency. See page 52.

Empty Heat – Another name for Yin Deficiency. See page 56.

Evil – A pathological influence that has invaded the body from the outside. See 'Wind' on page 68.

Jin Ye – Body fluids.

Jing – One of the '3 treasures' along with Qi and Shen. Jing, translated as 'Essence' is the deepest energy of the body, and forms the foundation for life. It is stored in the Kidneys. For Jing Deficiency, see page 58.

Jing Luo – The Chinese name for the network of channels or meridians.

Jue Yin – The name given to the pairing of the Liver and Pericardium channels. One of the 6 Divisions.

Meridian – A term for the pathways of Qi throughout the body. In this book, I use the term 'channel' instead. See page 106.

Nei Jing - One of the earliest books on Chinese medicine, still used today, full title 'Huang Di Nei Jing'.

Phlegm – A progression of Dampness. Involved in most chronic or complex conditions. See page 67.

Qi – One of the 3 Treasures, along with Jing and Shen. Qi is the energy that keeps you going from day to day. It is created out of food and air. For Qi Deficiency, see page 51.

Qi Gong – An alternate spelling of chi kung.

Qi Gong Tui Na - Another name for Yin style tui na. See page 116.

Ren – The Chinese name for the Conception Vessel. See page 106.

Replete – Used instead of 'excess' by some writers.

Retained Pathogen - If an external 'evil' invades the body, and is particularly strong, or the defensive Qi is very weak, it can penetrate more deeply, take hold, and becomes the start a chronic condition. This is called a 'retained pathogen'.

San Jiao – One of the 12 organs, which has 'a function but no form'. See page 88.

Shao Yang - The name given to the pairing of the Gall-Bladder and San Jiao channels. One of the 6 Divisions.

Shao Yin - The name given to the pairing of the Heart and Kidney channels. One of the 6 Divisions.

Shen – One of the 3 Treasures, along with Jing and Qi. Shen is often translated as 'Spirit' or 'Mind' and is to do with spirituality, mind and emotions. It is stored in the Heart – see page 82.

Shi – Chinese for 'excessive', sometimes used as a diagnostic term.

Shiatsu - The Japanese form of Qi-based bodywork, closely related to Chinese tui na.

T'ai Chi – A Chinese movement art, invaluable for self-cultivation and health maintenance. Also called t'ai chi ch'uan. See Chapter 11.

Tai Yang - The name given to the pairing of the Bladder and Small Intestine channels. One of the 6 Divisions.

Tai Yin - The name given to the pairing of the Lung and Spleen channels. One of the 6 Divisions.

Taiji – An alternate spelling of Tai Chi. Also called taiji chuan.

Tao – 'The Way'. See Taoism.

Taoism – An ancient Chinese philosophy, based around 'going with the flow' and following the way of nature.

TCM – Traditional Chinese Medicine. The standard form of Chinese Medicine practised worldwide. See page 16.

Tui Na – Literally 'push and grasp'. A Chinese massage therapy. See page 114.

Vacuous – Used instead of 'deficient' by some authors.

Wei Qi – Defensive Qi. Flows on the surface of the body, and defends against External Invasions.

Wind – External Wind refers to an 'invasion' of the body from the outside while Internal Wind refers to tics, tremors, shaking and convulsions and relates to the Liver. See pages 68 and 69.

Xu – Chinese for 'deficient', sometimes used as a diagnostic term.

Yang – One of the 2 primary poles of all existence – the so called 'male principle'. Yang is everything active, hot, moving, external and expansive. For Yang Deficiency, see page 52.

Yang Ming - The name given to the pairing of the Stomach and Large Intestine channels. One of the 6 Divisions.

Yin – One of the 2 primary poles of all existence – the so called 'female principle'. Yin is everything still, cold, quiet, internal and contracting. For Yin Deficiency, see page 56.

Ying Qi – Nutritive Qi. Flows inside the body, and nourishes the organs.

Zang Fu – The Chinese term for the organ system. The Zang are the Yin organs, which are solid and the Fu are the Yang organs, which are hollow.

Resources

The Author's Websites

The Radiant Health Blog – www.neilkingham.com
My personal site, for more information on all of the topics in this book and more. If you haven't already, I invite you to sign up for my free newsletter via the site, for all the latest information, and free gifts.

Qi Therapies – www.qi-therapies.com
The website for my Chinese Medicine clinic in the UK.

Further Reading

'The Web That Has No Weaver' – Ted Kaptchuk
A good introduction to Chinese medicine. Written for the lay-person, but very detailed. A good book if you're looking for a little more theory.

'The Chinese Massage Manual' – Sarah Pritchard
A great introduction to tui na massage by one of my teachers, and one the UK's leading experts on the subject.

'The Way Of Qi Gong' – Kenneth S Cohen
A lovely, detailed book on chi kung (Qi Gong) that describes

many of the differing approaches to this ancient art.

'Recipes For Self Healing' – Daverick Leggett
A fantastic easy to read book on Chinese Nutritional Therapy, with lots of recipes and a good introduction and background section.

'The Tao Of Healthy Eating' - Bob Flaws
Another good, accessible introduction to Chinese food energetics and dietary therapy

'The Ancient Wisdom Of The Chinese Tonic Herbs' - Ron Teeguarden
Detailed descriptions of the uses of tonic Chinese herbs for yang sheng purposes.

'Chinese Herbal Secrets' - Stefan Chmelik
A beautifully illustrated book, describing the principles of Chinese herbal medicine, and some of the most common herbs.

'The Tao Of Pooh' – Benjamin Hoff
A lovely introduction to Taoism. Very easy to read, and great fun.

Extra Free Resources

For further free resources related to this book, and to sign up for more information visit:

www.neilkingham.com/ugcm

Made in the USA
Charleston, SC
12 May 2014